RUNNING BEHIND

RUNNING BEHIND

Narratives of 40 Years Practicing Medicine

by

Richard K. Reed, M.D., F.A.C.P.

ISBN-13-9798629550044

Dedication

This book is dedicated to:

My loving wife

Connie Sue Reed,

My children

Jennifer Evin Reed Kelly, Jarrod Kyle Reed,

and Justin Richard Reed,

My grandchildren

Tucker Kyle Reed, Scarlett Llewellyn Kelly,

Sloane Isabella Reed, and Ryker Everett Reed

And

the thousands of patients from whom

I learned a great deal about life.

By Richard K. Reed, M.D., F.A.C.P.

Table of Contents

Dedication v

Foreword xi

Preface xiii

Chapter 1: The Case of Congestive Heart Failure: My Eyes Are Opened 1

Chapter 2: The Narrative of the Turkey Hunter 5

Chapter 3: Cardiac Resuscitation: Ethical or Unethical? 9

Chapter 4: The Patient with the Hard Heart 13

Chapter 5: Marked Money 17

Chapter 6: The Narrative of the Great Husband 19

Chapter 7: Facing Reality and the Cases of the Red Snappers 25

Chapter 8: The Tobacco Holocaust: A Call to Action 31

Chapter 9: The "Oh, by the Way" Diagnoses 37

Chapter 10: The Patient and His Bull 43

Chapter 11: The Missing Narratives: Cases of Poisoning 45

Chapter 12: An Unusual Case of Leg Pain 49

Chapter 13: Diagnostic and Therapeutic Dilemmas 53

Chapter 14: Dementia, the Sad Diagnosis....59

Chapter 15: Alcoholism: The Undiagnosed Disease....63

Chapter 16: The Missed Diagnoses: Lessons in Humility....69

Chapter 17: "The Queen"....75

Chapter 18: Miracles....79

Chapter 19: Frustrations in the Practice of Medicine: Acknowledging and Accepting Change....83

Chapter 20: Joys in Practicing Medicine: Home Visits....91

Chapter 21: Medicine of Tomorrow....95

Acknowledgements:

Justin R. Reed – Cover art and technical assistance

Connie S. Reed – Many hours of proofreading, editing, and typing

Linda McRae – Proofreading and editing

Foreword

In *Running Behind,* Richard Reed MD FACP reflects on a forty-year practice of internal medicine in northeast Tennessee. His collection of twenty-one narratives relate the joys and sorrows of his years of practice. He emphasizes the importance of clinical excellence, the necessity of making a correct diagnosis to provide proper patient care, and the value of listening to the patient to accomplish this. A man of faith, Dr. Reed discusses the spiritual aspects of care important for many of his patients. While sharing stories of success in making difficult diagnoses, Dr. Reed also shares experiences when errors occurred or proper diagnoses were not made. He shares some of the frustrations of the evolving practice of medicine. In his last chapter he offers guidelines for successful patient relationships to those considering health-related careers. Patients cared for by Dr. Reed were fortunate to have him as their physician. Medical students who worked with him were fortunate to have him as a role model. These accessible narratives are insightful, inspiring, and satisfying to read.

Kenneth E. Olive, MD MACP
Executive Associate Dean for Academic and Faculty Affairs
Professor of Internal Medicine
James H. Quillen College of Medicine, East Tennessee State University

Preface

Practicing medicine has been a wonderful blessing in my life. I have tried to be successful in helping people; in addition, I have also learned a great deal about life from these same people. My life has been enriched by developing relationships with them and being part of their life stories.

Below are a few goals for which I have written this book.

1. I hope that someone who reads it will decide on a medical or allied medical career.
2. My hope is that practitioners will be reminded of the relationship between faith and the practice of medicine.
3. My desire is that this book will help medical students, doctors in training, and young practicing physicians to understand the value - to themselves and their patients - of seeing the humanity in their patients in their present situation and in their future practices. Hopefully, practitioners will be better able to deal with their present or future stress and burnout when they begin seeing patients as people, rather than just their disease. I believe that the lives of the doctors will be enriched by the stories they hear from their patients when they spend the extra time needed to hear those stories.
4. I hope the book will help lay people get some idea of how doctors can relate to patients and their diseases.

Running behind was always on my mind in my 41 years and 3 months in the practice of medicine. With almost every patient I saw in the office or hospital, running behind with my schedule of patients always bothered me. I did not like the patients to wait on me anymore than I like to wait on someone else. Somewhere in my medical training, I learned that patients do not mind waiting up to twenty minutes. Beyond that, they can become annoyed. In the busiest years of practice, I worked at two hospitals and one office. Occasionally, afternoon patients would have to wait up to forty-five minutes or longer to see me. I learned to apologize to all of them – even if I was late by only ten minutes or so.

Whether or not I was on time, spending quality time with the patients by listening to all of their complaints and doing a careful examination each time seemed to translate into a good visit. It also showed concern, developed rapport, and led to historical and physical examination findings that might have been missed otherwise. It also built a sense of trust in our doctor-patient relationship. This trust became a solid foundation on which lasting relationships were built. Running behind and then getting a late start with the next patient was no excuse for spending less quality time with *that* patient. It was not worth the risk of making a wrong diagnosis or not building that strong relationship with the patient.

Unfortunately, the emphasis of healthcare systems on providers is seeing larger numbers of patients in order to increase the income of the system; this results in limited face-to-face time with patients. How can the kind of relationship that was just discussed possibly be developed with as little as fifteen minutes of face-to-face time with the patient?

The narratives in the chapters that follow demonstrate relationships that grew stronger with time, based on my attempt to spend adequate, quality time with each patient. These relationships began by seeing patients as persons of worth, not just patients with a particular disease. In addition, this book is not just about me; it is not an autobiography. The true message is about the humanity of my patients. Their diseases proved to be a conduit for developing a doctor-patient relationship that hopefully made as much of a difference in their lives as it did in mine. From my standpoint, these relationships made me a different and better person as well as a more appreciative physician.

The patients and their stories are real. However, their names, places of origin, and occupations are fictitious. I have also changed some of the details about their illnesses to disguise their identity.

Without realizing it at the time, my high school, college, and medical school education along with my residency training would guide my thinking through a 41-year practice of medicine. I had no idea that the thousands of scholastic and practical experiences I had would culminate in the writing of this book in my retirement. These experiences, discussed in the body of this book, made me the physician I am today. I chose medicine as a career because of my interest in the science of biology associated with the human body. Mr. James M. Phillips (his real name), my high school biology teacher at Morristown High School in Morristown, Tennessee, had a tremendous influence on my becoming a doctor and on my life in general. He gave me more than information about biology. He gave me encouragement to pursue my dreams. Without his influence, I would likely never have become a physician.

A love for learning followed me into college and medical school. In medical school, I chose internal medicine as my career path and subsequent residency. At the University of Tennessee Medical Units in Memphis, Tennessee, I was fortunate to have Dr. Gene Stollerman, the Chief of the medicine department, as my mentor for four and a half years. Because Dr. Stollerman emphasized the *scientific* aspects of medicine, I learned the significance of applying accurate scientific inquiry as opposed to just opinion or anecdotal experiences. He emphasized, "The more science – the better the medicine."

Dr. Stollerman's approach to medicine was the primacy of patient care. From him, I learned that the patient's history and physical examinations are the most important part of the doctor-patient relationship. These examinations can ultimately lead to the patient's correct diagnosis if adequate time is spent and the information gleaned is viewed through a scientific lens. Dr. Stollerman's emphasis in medicine was to always make the right diagnosis. The right diagnosis is the starting point of all good physicians' work. After the thorough examination of the patient, the correct diagnosis sets the stage for treatment plans such as surgery, medications, physical therapy, occupational therapy, radiation therapy, etc. But first, the right diagnosis must be made!

The physician should always view the patient's visit as a privilege and as a compliment for being chosen as the one to help them with their healthcare. People want to be seen as people, not just a number or a click on a computer screen. My hope is that this book will highlight patients as people and will help future practitioners keep humanity in the practice of medicine.

The good physician treats the disease;
the great physician treats the patient who has the disease."

— Sir William Osler

Chapter 1

The Case of Congestive Heart Failure: My Eyes Are Opened

"...for the secret of the care of the patient is in caring for the patient."

— Francis W. Peabody

Sam Brown came from West Memphis, Arkansas, to see me during my internship at the VA Hospital in Memphis, Tennessee while I was in training at the University of Tennessee. Our service, called the house staff team, cared for him. The team was comprised of four medical students, two interns, and one medicine resident. We also had an attending physician from the VA or general medical community with whom we made rounds four times per week.

Mr. Brown had come to the hospital because of shortness of breath which is generally caused by diseases of the heart, lungs, or blood. I learned in medical school that shortness of breath is the hardest symptom in medicine to diagnose. Mr. Brown was found to have systolic congestive heart failure. As a result, his heart was failing in its job of pumping blood to the brain, kidneys, and other vital organs. This inefficiency of the heart's pumping action resulted in blood and fluid backing up in his lungs, which is why he became short of breath. The alveoli (air sacs) in the lung were filled with fluid rather than air. He responded well to intravenous furosemide, a diuretic that caused excretion of the fluid through his kidneys and out of his body. As a result, his shortness of breath improved.

His faithful son always tended to Mr. Brown. Before he left the hospital, Mr. Brown and his son thanked me greatly for his care. His son asked if his father could come back to see me in my clinic, a half day per week when patients were seen as a follow-up to their hospitalization. Only residents, not interns, had "clinics," so I told him that I would get him an appointment with our house staff team resident. However, both Mr. Brown and his son were insistent that they see me. I was very flattered by their request. When they came back to see me in the house staff office in the hospital a couple of weeks later, he was much better.

I felt an incredible sense of accomplishment! I had correctly diagnosed his congestive heart failure and treated him appropriately, but there was more to the story. By spending time with Mr. Brown, I had "connected" with both the patient and his son. I had developed rapport, which engendered an atmosphere of mutual trust. This patient and his son knew that I had their best interests at heart. This was my moment of epiphany. My eyes were opened to the patient as a person – not just a patient with a disease and not just another case of congestive heart failure.

I recognized that I had communicated with him in a way that I had not communicated with a patient previously

About a year later while practicing medicine in the U.S. Navy, I had a great experience with another patient. This became my second epiphany moment. Capt. Jackson Caroli Merriweather was retired from the Navy and lived in Inyokern, California. He had graduated from the U.S. Naval Academy in 1931 and later served as a senior naval officer in WWII during which he saw duty in the North Atlantic. In 1955, he retired early as Executive officer at the local Navy base in order to care for his mother. He had high blood pressure and frequent premature ventricular contractions (extra heartbeats that originated from the left ventricle).

He saw a cardiologist in our local Ridgecrest, California area who treated him. Although he also saw a civilian general practitioner in town, he always came back to me at the dispensary on the Navy base. He developed trust in me as a Navy physician.

A long-time bachelor, Capt. Merriweather hosted my wife and me several evenings in his high desert home to have dinner, enjoy his "wine coolers," and watch the mail plane coming into Ridgecrest from Los Angeles. The rapport we developed made us feel more comfortable around each other. Capt. Merriweather even told me that he would give me some of his land near his home on which I could build a medical office. I thanked him but decided against it. This relationship confirmed for me that in the future I wanted to practice medicine with the patient, not the patient's disease as the focal point.

With these experiences, I also recognized a trait that I had been using without realizing it – empathy. Working with these patients helped me to recognize that I had probably always had empathy but just was not aware of it.

The most noted physician who wrote of empathy was Francis Weld Peabody. Known for his research into poliomyelitis and typhoid, he was a celebrated teacher at the Harvard Medical School. He wrote "The Care of the Patient" which initially appeared in the Journal of the American Medical Association in 1927. The quote at the beginning of this chapter is his statement about empathy.

These patient encounters followed me throughout my next four decades of medical practice. After developing rapport with them, I began to see every person in my office not just as a patient in need of a diagnosis, treatment, and follow-up but as a human being; I saw their humanity. Their humanity rose above the *science* of medicine which only sees people through the lens of their diseases. In addition, I learned something that would help me years later. Getting to know people on a personal level would help me to deal with the stresses of practicing medicine and help to quell burnout that would come with years of practicing. My experiences with Mr. Brown and his son as well as Capt. Merriweather did put me behind in seeing my next patient. I learned early on that perhaps running behind would help me in developing relationships with patients.

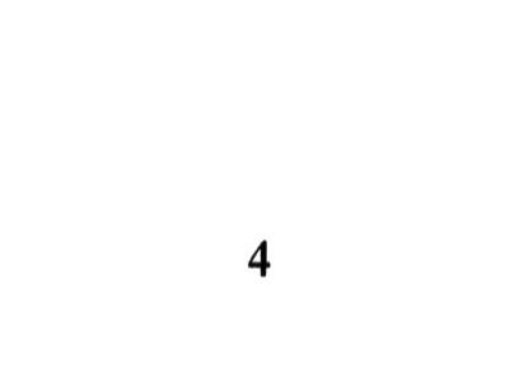

Chapter 2

The Narrative of the Turkey Hunter

"Physicians need rhetoric as much as knowledge, and they need stories as much as journals if they are to be more sympathetic than computers."

— Howard Spiro, M.D.

When I first heard of the *narrative* in medicine, I had no idea what it meant. Following a discussion about its purpose and benefits at an internal medicine conference, I realized that many physicians, including me, had been using it for years.

The narrative helps the doctor to get to know the patient and the family better, thereby helping him to build a bond with the patient. The classic example of the narrative lies in the relationship of pastor or priest to parishioner. The bond is formed by a relationship of mutual respect, trust (including confidentiality), admiration, and a genuine willingness to give honest advice to improve the parishioner's or patient's life. I always felt that the physician should care for his patients as a pastor cares for his parishioners – like a shepherd to his flock.

Mr. Thomas Sherrill was a man with a strong faith in Christ. He worked as an accountant. One of his colleagues told me that because of Mr. Sherill's vast accounting experience, he was one of the most respected professionals in his workplace.

He developed several medical problems. As a result of having pulmonary emboli (blood clots to the lungs) years before, he was on anticoagulants (blood thinners). He *also* had high blood pressure. In addition, he had developed interstitial lung disease, or scarring in his lungs, the cause of which was unknown. He had no known occupational exposure at his workplace that would have explained the lung disease. Finally, he had a new diagnosis of cancer.

Sarah, his wife, was also my patient. She, too, also had cancer and a predisposition to infections. Until a correct diagnosis of a suppressed immune system was made, she had frequent bouts of sinusitis and bronchitis. Mr. Sherrill's main concern was for Sarah's health, in spite of his own most severe problem – worsening interstitial lung disease. During the latter years of his life, he was on continuous oxygen. In order to get him to smile, I only had to mention his wife or his favorite pastime – turkey hunting. He hunted nothing but turkey. An avid gun person, the only guns he owned were for turkey hunting.

He was particularly worried about his wife with her recurrent infections and repeated hospitalizations. Following one of these hospitalizations and before he himself was on oxygen, he found time to go turkey hunting. On a particular hunt in the fall, he found a gobbler that he thought would look good on their Thanksgiving table. He told me how he raised his shotgun for the kill. As he continued the story, he looked at me with tears in his eyes. He said that he did not fire the fatal shot. In fact, he did not fire the gun at all. He said that his thoughts at that moment were, "I'll let this gobbler live and hope that God, in turn, will let my wife live." He left the woods that day *without* a turkey but *with* a heart full of love for his wife and his God. While there were few times in the office when I shed tears with a patient, this was the most memorable time of all.

As alluded to in the Preface, I dislike the standard fifteen-minute appointments for patients. However, I did not have to worry about this with Mr. Sherrill. He usually just showed up at the office without an appointment or called me on my cell phone instead of going through the office phone. At first, these behaviors were aggravating. In time, though, I grew to admire him so much that I no longer saw his unscheduled visits and phone calls as a nuisance.

One day, Mr. Sherrill came into the office unexpectedly with his wife for what turned out to be his final office visit. The purpose for the visit was his wife's cough and shortness of breath, which I diagnosed as pneumonia. I insisted that he be examined as well since his respiratory state appeared to be even worse than hers was. Resistant at first, he succumbed to my questions and examination. Both spouses were diagnosed with pneumonia and had to be hospitalized. He refused to go by ambulance, so he called his pastor who kindly took them both to the hospital. While Mrs. Sherrill was discharged from the hospital in only a few days, her husband, unfortunately, did not survive. The lung infection superimposed on his interstitial lung disease was too much for him. Though he eventually lost the battle, his turkey hunt had been successful - Sarah was doing well.

His unexpected phone calls and office visits always put me behind with my roster of patients. However, now I just remember the good visits I had with Mr. Sherrill. This time, running behind had been good medicine for my own life.

Chapter 3

Cardiac Resuscitation: Ethical or Unethical?

"Ethics are more important than laws."

— Wynton Marsalis

Bertha Hatfield was an elderly lady who had at least moderate cognitive impairment (dementia). I had done an MMSE (Mini Mental Status Examination) on her. This is a bedside tool that allows physicians to assign a number to a patient's cognitive ability. It is a screening tool only and does not make a definitive diagnosis of dementia. A perfect score is 30. She scored 18. This low score, when considered in the light of her total clinical picture, placed her in the category of at least moderate dementia.

Her other medical problems included longstanding hypertension as well as hypertensive heart disease. This means that she, at least, had left ventricular hypertrophy. Hypertrophy is a thickening of the heart muscle which can eventually cause the heart to lose its pumping ability, resulting in congestive heart failure. When Mrs. Hatfield came to the hospital with symptoms of shortness of breath and fatigue, she was found to have congestive heart failure (CHF). With proper treatment, she improved.

Mrs. Hatfield's two loving daughters were usually at her side or were discussing their mother's health with me by phone. This was especially true in regards to her mental status. One Sunday morning while making rounds in the hospital, I entered her room and noticed that one of her sons-in-law was there but the daughters were conspicuously absent. When I asked how she was doing, Mrs. Hatfield smiled and told me that she felt much better. With the help of a social worker, arrangements were made for her to go to a nursing home for convalescence and rehabilitation, at least temporarily. I assumed that her daughters were consulted about this. She was ready to be discharged but, as yet, had not been disconnected from her cardiac monitor via telemetry.

As I continued to talking with Mrs. Hatfield, she suddenly lost consciousness. The monitor showed ventricular tachycardia, an abnormal rhythm that can lead to ventricular fibrillation and death. At that moment, I could not remember her code status which refers to the status of a patient as to whether or not a patient should be resuscitated with cardiopulmonary resuscitation (CPR), electrical defibrillation and even intubation of the trachea (the process of placing a tube down the throat and into the windpipe.) It is generally best not to resuscitate a patient who has severe dementia. Even knowing that I *must* have had a discussion with her daughters about their wishes for their mother's code status, I could not remember that discussion. In the daughters' absence, I looked to the son-in-law. He just shrugged his shoulders when asked about CPR.

Mrs. Hatfield was unconscious and pulseless with an unstable ventricular rhythm on the EKG monitor. I knew that ventricular tachycardia would often respond to the "precordial thump" which can generate around five joules of electrical current, but I also knew that it was out of vogue with current recommendations on CPR from the American Heart Association. Nevertheless, I made the decision to administer the precordial thump, and she responded nicely. The monitor showed that a regular rhythm had been restored, she had a strong pulse, and her blood pressure had come up. More importantly, she awoke and smiled. The following day she was discharged to the nursing home. On the third day of her recuperation in the nursing home, Mrs. Hatfield died.

She must have had an episode of ventricular fibrillation. Except for a beta-blocker, she had not been discharged on medication to prevent more heart rhythm problems. No repeat echocardiograms were done to look at heart function to determine the potential benefit of an implantable defibrillator that can save the patient's life by shocking the heart when a potentially serious rhythm problem is detected Over the next two days after the cardiac resuscitation, I felt guilty. It felt as though I had violated some ethical law of behavior for physicians. This was especially true when I discovered later that Mrs. Hatfield's daughters had, in fact, approved a "No Code" status for their mother.

After her mother's death, one of her daughters called me at the office. I told her that I was sorry about her mother's sudden death and about resuscitating her in the hospital. Her daughter's next comment was a huge surprise! She thanked me profusely for having revived her mother. She said that the family had talked with her for years about her faith. She would never commit her life to the Lord. However, during her last three days in the nursing home, she finally made her profession of faith in Christ. The daughter was not just delighted; she was tearfully delighted.

I believe that ethical treatment was given to Mrs. Hatfield. In addition, I know *Where* she is today. Mrs. Hatfield took a lot of my time both in the hospital and in the office. I ran behind seeing my next patients. However, in this case, running behind was *Heavenly* spent.

Chapter 4

The Patient with the Hard Heart

"The Heart moves of itself and does not stop, unless forever."

— Leonardo da Vinci

Calvin Goodgame was an unusual patient. Everyone in our office who had interacted with him dreaded his arrival. He became notoriously known as the dreaded patient. However, at each visit he entered the office with a smile. This was his best trait. Despite his smile, his appearance in the office portended a visit of complaining, sarcasm, and even hostility. He was not able to sit in our waiting room without evoking the ire of other patients. He hated Republicans, George Bush, and the medical profession in general. He seemed to relish provoking arguments, especially about politics. There were times when the nurses in the office threatened to call security. Yet, despite these shortcomings, there seemed to be something about him that gave familiarity to the first syllable of his last name. Perhaps it was that initial smile? However, once the English language came forth from his mouth, his true nature revealed itself.

I tried to develop better rapport with him by spending extra time with him, calling him at home and even visiting him there. He did not listen to suggestions to cultivate friendships, go to the Senior Center, attend church, volunteer at the hospital (good luck!), or do something to make him happier in his retirement years. Even though I did my best to soften his hard heart, my efforts were not the least bit successful.

In addition, he liked to convey a sense of intellectual superiority. It seemed that he had always wanted to be known as a person with a scientific background. His area of work, though, was unrelated to science.

One day on entering his examining room, he told me about his son being an architect. His derogatory comment that followed was that his son made a lot of money as an architect but never, of course, as much as "you doctors". His comments always *preceded* my probing medical history and examinations. On this day, he was proceeding to explain to me about the function of the adrenal glands which sit on top of each kidney and regulate blood pressure, cortisol, sodium, potassium, and certain hormones in the blood. While I actually appreciated his insight into the functioning of the body in general, he was way off base with regard to his own medical problems.

He had several medical problems, including hypertension, diabetes, arthritis of his knee, and, importantly, aortic stenosis, a common form of aortic valve disease. This condition occurs when calcium builds up in the aortic valve through which blood flows from the left ventricle into the aorta. The aortic valve normally prevents blood pumped out of the ventricle from simply re-entering the ventricle following systole (the forceful contraction of the left ventricle). When the valve becomes heavily calcified, however, this function is impeded. The patient develops symptoms of progressive shortness of breath, syncope (fainting, or a feeling of faintness), near syncope, swelling in the legs, and angina (chest pressure or tightness brought on by physical activity or exertion and relieved by rest).

Mr. Goodgame had many of these symptoms. He was eventually referred to a well-respected cardiovascular surgeon in our community who recommended an open chest surgical procedure to replace his aortic valve. This was before the days of TAVR, or transcatheter aortic valve replacement, which obviates the need for an open chest procedure. TAVR involves placing a catheter or tube into a large artery in the leg in order to access the aortic valve, followed by replacement of the valve.

Following the procedure, the surgeon called me to report that upon opening the patient's chest, he found that the patient's aorta was very hard, like an eggshell. Because of this "porcelainized" aorta, the operation could not be performed, and his chest was closed without the planned and necessary valve replacement.

On returning to see me in the office, he had a scar on his chest but no new heart valve. We discussed his problem, including his scientific knowledge of aortic valve disease in general.

He was then referred to a large university medical center. A different procedure for aortic valve replacement was attempted there. Unfortunately, Mr. Goodgame died a few days later of postoperative complications.

As usual, I called his family following his death. His daughter told me that he had no funeral service. Apparently, a nonbeliever, he was also buried with no graveside service. She said that he had no friends which explained the reason that the only ones in attendance at his burial were his architect son and his nurse daughter.

It is possible for a patient to have "healing without curing." This is generally realized by physicians only after many years of practicing medicine. This is not something one necessarily learns in medical school or residency. Unfortunately, in the case of Mr. Goodgame, I am not sure if either healing *or* curing had taken place.

Working with Mr. Goodgame taught me to develop a passion for working with difficult patients – especially for those who are suspicious of the medical profession. As a fellow human interacting with this man, I tried to follow the advice of an unknown author who said, "Be kind to unkind people. They need it the most."

Just running behind was not a problem with this patient. I always ran *far* behind after seeing him. I do have some regrets about not healing *or* curing his "hard heart." emotionally and physically. However, I do have one good memory about him as a person. His smile, even today, seemed heartfelt to me. Perhaps it was a clue to a hidden secret locked in his subconscious waiting to be opened and explored by a more skilled clinician.

I will never know. However, this I do know – he gave *me healing* in my attitude about taking care of difficult patients

Chapter 5

Marked Money

"We are here to add what we can to life, not to get what we can from life."

— Sir William Osler

Fred Robertson was a very large man with a jovial personality. Up in years, he had become quite successful financially. Except for mild cognitive impairment (dementia), hypertension, and obesity, he had been fairly healthy. When he developed symptoms of fever and shortness of breath, he came to the hospital emergency department. After viewing his x-ray, he was diagnosed with pneumonia. However, the chest x-ray also revealed something else; there was fluid in his left lung. On examination, he had some respiratory distress in addition to his fever. Another concern was that his white blood cell count was very high at 35,000. White blood cells fight infection; a normal white blood cell count is 5,000-10,000. It was felt that the fluid on his lung could be purulence (pus), which could possibly explain his elevated white blood cells. Therefore, a thoracentesis was undertaken by inserting a needle through the chest wall to aspirate fluid. The fluid was indeed purulent. This demonstrated that he did in fact have pneumonia, but with the complication of an "empyema" (fluid *around* the lung that has become secondarily infected from the pneumonia). A low pH (pointing to acidity) on this fluid also pointed to the fact that he needed a chest tube to drain the fluid. A chest tube is a large bore tube inserted to facilitate continuous drainage and removal of the pus. He did well with the chest tube placement as well as intravenous fluids, oxygen, and antibiotics. After about ten days in the hospital, he was discharged with no fever. He made a good, complete recovery from a very serious illness and seemed to be left without serious sequella of any lung disease.

When I saw him for follow-up in the office in the many years following this illness, he was always very appreciative of the care he had received. He always made a special effort to thank me.

Mr. Robertson usually wore a large plaid shirt over a white t-shirt. The shirt had a large, open, right-sided pocket. At the end of each visit, he would reach down into this pocket and pull out a $100 bill. As he handed it to me, he would wink and say, "Dr. Reed, I appreciate your services so much." I noticed that the $100 bill had a red star drawn on the obverse side. The star was quite large and obvious. During the visit, I would direct his attention to the left as I proceeded with the customary physical examination. As he would look to the left, I quickly placed the marked bill back into his large, open, right-sided shirt pocket. None the wiser, he left the office with the $100 bill still in his possession. Over the years, he paid me with many extra $100 bills – albeit the *same* marked bill.

Mr. Robertson always appreciated my services to him. Likewise, I always appreciated seeing and caring for Mr. Robertson as well.

My memories of this patient are always as pleasant as seeing his smiling face. The relationship of the physician and patient in this case was far more rewarding than any denominations of money.

I spent extra time with Mr. Robertson at each of his visits. As a result, I was always running behind. Perhaps the next patient visit would bring even more challenges. Running behind was not really so bad after all.

Chapter 6

The Narrative of the Great Husband

"A good husband wipes her tears but a great husband listens to the story of why she is crying."

— Author Unknown

Mr. Robert Holbrook was a devoted husband to his wife Phyllis. Although in his early 60's, he looked to be around 50 years old. By training, his job was very technical; he was very practical, and had a lot of common sense, which he called "street smarts". He was able to fix just about anything, but automobiles were his forte.

As an electrical engineer, Mr. Holbrook had worked on the Apollo project that sent man to the moon. While he was involved in Apollo 4 through Apollo 11, he felt his contribution to the latter, Apollo 11, was his most important. This project resulted in Neil Armstrong and Buzz Aldrin being the first humans to walk on the moon. He was in charge of eleven hundred measurements on the launch pad facility, including the crawler-transporter that carried the Apollo 11 Saturn 5 rocket from the VAB (Vehicle Assembly Building) to Launch Pad 39A from where it was launched to the moon. The gauges included sensors for pressure, wind speed (anemometer), hydrogen, oxygen, and fire. The point to be made is that his knowledge of the practical and technical aspects of engineering allowed him to be involved in one of the most well-known scientific feats in the history of mankind. He never knew how important this knowledge would be to his family in the future!

When Phyllis came to see me after developing headaches, I evaluated her and eventually referred her to a neurologist and then to a neurosurgeon. She was found to have a brain aneurysm. Surgery was recommended. At the time of surgery, a lot of bleeding occurred from an apparent rupture of the aneurysm. Because of this rupture, part of the cerebellum had to be removed. The cerebellum is at the back of the brain, makes up about ten percent of its total weight, and plays the important role of coordinating voluntary movements such as posture, balance, coordination, and speech. Its function results in smooth and coordinated muscular movement. After surgery, her neurologic status caused her to change from a vibrant family and businesswoman to a patient with severe disabilities, unable to live as she had previously.

Phyllis was also unable to breathe on her own due to the neurologic damage. She was in the intensive care unit on a ventilator, a machine to maintain breathing, or ventilation of the lungs and oxygenation of the blood. Oxygenation of the blood refers to maintaining the right amount of oxygen in the blood for normal human functioning. Being unable to breathe on her own without the ventilator became Phyllis' primary problem.

In his quest to help her, Robert became convinced that he would be able to get her off the ventilator. He began to work with the respiratory therapists and pulmonary doctors (lung specialists) to learn as much as he could about the physical aspects of her situation. He learned about the normal ventilation mechanism that all of us have – the "sigh." The sigh is an involuntary action or signal which comes from the brainstem – the part of the brain that regulates breathing and heart function. The sigh helps to ventilate all portions of the lungs equally to improve overall ventilation and oxygenation. By listening carefully to her breathing, Robert discovered that Phyllis would sigh on her own without the sigh originating from the respirator! Using his common sense, he assumed that this meant that she had some brain function that could possibly help her in getting off the ventilator. In addition, when he asked her to take a deep breath on her own, she did it without mechanical ventilator assistance at all!

He continued to stay with Phyllis day and night. He did much more than that, though! Remember the eleven hundred gauges that he was in charge of while working as an engineer on the Apollo project? He was about to put his expertise to good use for Phyllis.

After becoming familiar with the ventilator by working in concert with the respiratory therapist, he helped Phyllis make progress in her breathing when he started handling the ventilator controls himself. Eventually, the pulmonary doctor had instructed the floor nurses to "let Robert handle all the respiratory controls." After a period of time, a miracle happened! Phyllis was taken off the ventilator, and she could breathe on her own! Robert's understanding of and comfort with working with gauges ended up benefiting his wife immensely. The nursing staff was amazed at Mr. Holbrook's tenacity. Initially they had concerns about a patient's spouse being around constantly and being so involved in the functioning of the ventilator. By the end of her stay there, they considered him a friend and "colleague". One nurse reported to me that her own husband was a good husband. However, after knowing Robert Holbrook she told me that she had learned the qualities of a "great" husband. I have never witnessed such good caregiving by a family member.

Even though Phyllis had made great progress, she still had a long way to go in terms of physical and occupational therapy. In addition, she was "locked in" because of her brain injury. The "locked-in" syndrome (LIS), or pseudocoma, is a condition in which the patient is aware but cannot communicate this awareness verbally.

She was transferred to a rehabilitation facility near Boston, MA. One of her needs was to regain her ability to communicate, so the doctors told Robert that he needed to communicate more with his wife. While he had been doing this, he followed the doctors' orders and started working more diligently on his communication with Phyllis. She soon became better able to respond to commands and eventually it was clear that she knew the alphabet. Robert also worked with the physical and occupational therapists to increase her abilities in these areas as well. Eventually, she moved from the bed to a chair. On one occasion while sitting in her chair, she had some chest pain. While she could not say "EKG," she did communicate "electrocardiogram" by softly speaking each letter of the word so they knew of her condition.

The rehabilitation doctor in Boston was very impressed with Mr. Holbrook. In fact, the doctor asked Robert to call him when she left the hospital. When he called the doctor, he told Robert something he had never said to any other caregiver. He said, "I learned something from you." The doctor told Robert that he had learned that tenacious, loving care can result in wondrous medical benefits. Needless to say, I learned something, too.

Always wanting the best care for his wife, he then moved her to a rehabilitation center in Florida, and eventually back to their home. Robert worked with her so hard that eventually she was able to walk with help! Sadly, she later died from respiratory failure.

Mr. Holbrook was indeed a remarkable person. His technical expertise, combined with common sense, his tenacity, and his loving concern for his spouse all added up to a medical miracle. While she never experienced complete recovery, she definitely did not die for nothing. In the process of caring for her before her death, the lives of many people were touched – her physicians, therapists, nurses, and family members. Also, the medical community learned much by being involved in her care and in their association with her husband, Robert Holbrook. In 1867, the famous physician, Oliver Wendell Holmes, said, "The most essential part of a student's instruction is obtained, as I believe, not in the lecture room, but at the bedside." The bed of Phyllis Holbrook resulted in many medical care providers gaining advanced degrees in tenacity and loving care.

Mr. Holbrook had always been a man of faith. He had been involved in one of the greatest achievements of aviation in sending man to the heavens. In caring for his wife, his own soul was heaven directed as well.

Seeing Mrs. Holbrook resulted in a lot of time being spent with the patient and her husband. Running behind with my schedule was again a constant reminder of the many demands of a medical practice. However, in this case, I learned a great deal about humanity and the practice of medicine. I learned about the importance of having an advocate for your healthcare needs. In the days of medical marketing, tight schedules of patients for providers, and the demand for making money, an advocate is a top priority, especially when you cannot be the advocate for your own health.

Chapter 7

Facing Reality and the Cases of the Red Snappers

"Nothing becomes more real until it is experienced – even a proverb is no proverb until your life has illustrated it."

—John Keats

John Keats was my favorite Romantic poet in high school in Morristown, Tennessee in the 1960s. I once did a Senior English paper on his famous "Ode on a Grecian Urn." I learned a great deal about English literature, the Romantic poets, and life in general from this assignment.

Learning how to help patients face reality was always a challenge for me. *Accepting* bad news is always tough but *giving* bad news is hard as well. Most cases of bad news involve a diagnosis of cancer. News about ostensibly incurable cancer is always particularly hard. People do react differently to bad news. Some patients respond with tears and depression. Many have an attitude of "I will beat this disease." A good positive attitude can go a long way to help a patient fight a poor diagnosis.

I once again review the admonition of my mentor Dr. Gene Stollerman at the University of Tennessee Medical Units in Memphis, "Making the correct diagnosis is the most important gift we can give a patient."

My wife, Connie, and I had to face reality when our middle son was about fifteen months old. He had had fever for approximately five weeks. The pediatrician kept giving him antibiotics for ear infections. Our son was eventually hospitalized and was found to have an enlarged spleen. He subsequently had positive blood cultures. He was diagnosed with endocarditis, an infection on a heart valve. Specifically, his aortic valve was infected. It was felt that he likely had a congenital defect with a bicuspid aortic valve. The aortic valve normally has three cusps, or parts, but apparently, his had only two. He later developed aortic insufficiency (leakage caused by incompetent valve function). In his teenage years, he had to have two heart surgeries with the latter one being replacement of his aortic valve. The shock of our son having endocarditis was overwhelming for both Connie and me. We learned to cope with our frustration and fears through the years though. Prayer was a large part of our coping strategy!

Having to face the reality of serious illness in my own family made me a better physician. I had personally experienced the value of a correct diagnosis. A good doctor sees patients as human beings with a disease rather than a disease in some nameless person. William Osler's statement that, "The good physician treats the disease; the great physician treats the patient who has the disease" had become reality and changed my life forever.

Of course, receiving a diagnosis of cancer seems to be the one that is most feared. However, cancer is by no means the only diagnosis about which patients have to face harsh reality. My own son's experience is one example of that. I distinctly remember four cases in my years of practice where reality meant facing death head on. These cases were associated with infections rather than cancer.

Mr. John W. Shaw was from neighboring Lee County, Virginia. His history revealed that he had lost weight, with a bad cough, some fever, and sweating at night. His chest x-ray showed evidence of an abnormality in the right upper lobe of his lung. Having seen him in the hospital setting, I reviewed his x-rays with the radiologist. With his weight loss and cough along with a smoking history, lung cancer was high on the differential diagnostic list. I took some early morning collected sputum for culture to look for granulomatous disease, including tuberculosis. Granulomatous diseases include TB and fungal diseases such as histoplasmosis which is common in the Ohio and Mississippi river valleys, blastomycosis, and coccidioidomycosis, the latter of which is common in the Western U.S. deserts. (I had seen cases of Valley fever or coccidioidomycosis while in California in the Navy.)

I asked one of our local pathologists to review the sputum stains for acid fast bacilli, which include TB, or Mycobacterium tuberculosis. We both looked at them for a total of three hours one day. Low and behold, one of us finally shouted, "Red snappers!" We had found tiny bacteria that stain red on a blue field when a particular stain is used. First described by Koch in 1882, we had found the bacteria and diagnosed my first presumptive case of tuberculosis in Kingsport. We reported this case to the local health department and started him on anti-tuberculosis therapy. He was placed in isolation in the hospital during his treatment. HIV, often associated with TB, was not around at that time and, as a result, was not something about which we were concerned. Later his culture did grow Mycobacterium tuberculosis. While red snappers can indicate other diseases, including leprosy, a positive culture establishes a firm diagnosis of tuberculosis.

Initially, Mr. Shaw and his family had a hard time accepting this diagnosis, even though it had a much better cure rate than lung cancer. Facing the reality of the red snappers, he eventually discovered he was lucky, or "blessed." I favor the latter designation.

Mr. Jessie Homer Johnson was in his 80s when I first saw him for examination. He seemed to be healthy overall for his age except for high blood pressure. One day I was in the grocery store and saw him. We greeted each other. Then he began complaining of a cough and shortness of breath. I asked him to come to the office for examination. As my nurse escorted him down the hall to the examining room, he coughed up a large amount of green colored sputum. Immediately I had the sputum sent for staining and cultures. That afternoon the microbiology lab called me and reported that "red snappers" were seen on the stains. He was hospitalized, isolated, and started on antituberculous therapy. When his sputums were negative for active tuberculi bacilli, he was sent home. Five weeks later, his culture grew Mycobacterium tuberculosis.

Interestingly, a few weeks later, I again saw him in public – this time at a local bank. He told me that he had been doing well until two weeks prior when he had developed shortness of breath, chest pain, and had coughed some blood. Resistant T.B. was my first thought. In the office the next day he was examined. Particular imaging studies were performed that confirmed a diagnosis of pulmonary emboli – blood clots in the lungs. Perhaps the origin of his blood clots was from his legs, having developed at the time of his hospitalization for TB when he was at bedrest for some time. He was started on anticoagulant therapy as he also continued his therapy for tuberculosis. A few weeks later, I once again saw him in public. This time he was once again back in the grocery store. From a distance, he did not look to be short of breath.

Mr. Johnson had to face harsh reality twice with TB and blood clots in the lungs. A man of God, he faced both problems with grace and dignity. This time I was the one who felt blessed to have cared for him.

Dr. Sam Richardson was an endocrinology fellow in training at the University of Tennessee. As a general internal medicine fellow, I saw him in the clinic one day for a chronic cough. A chest x-ray showed a surprising finding. He appeared to have a "miliary" pattern on the chest x-ray suggestive of tuberculosis. He underwent a lung biopsy that proved to be TB. Anti-tuberculous therapy had already been instituted. As a doctor, he was shocked to have active tuberculosis.

Mrs. Alice Cromwell had presented with back pain. Imaging studies showed evidence of a lytic lesion (like a hole) in a lumbar vertebra in her spine. She had also had a positive PPD, a skin test used to diagnose the presence of the tuberculi bacillus in the human body. However, it cannot distinguish active disease from dormant disease or from previous exposure to TB. A biopsy of the vertebral lesion yielded findings consistent with active tuberculosis (Pott's disease). She also was treated with anti-tuberculous therapy. She was quite surprised that she came out of the hospital with tuberculosis when her only complaint was back pain. However, she did accept reality and took her therapy.

Other physicians NOT making a diagnosis of tuberculosis have had to face their own reality as well. After being hit by a car in the 1960s, a female patient was admitted to a famous hospital. As part of her work up, a bone marrow examination was done that showed findings consistent with aplastic anemia, a situation in which the bone marrow simply stops making blood for no known reason. She sought treatment from many famous doctors, including those at Columbia-Presbyterian Hospital in New York City. Her doctors started her on steroids (Prednisone) for her aplastic anemia. When she then developed a fever, blood work was done that showed her sedimentation rate was markedly elevated at 128. The sedimentation rate is a blood test that is very sensitive but not specific for certain diseases, including infections. To the surprise of her doctors, with more extensive investigation, the patient was found to have tuberculosis. On reflection, the anemia was most likely due to tuberculosis from the start. The patient being discussed was Eleanor Roosevelt; she died at the age of 78.

There is a prominent person who was quoted about the true nature of experiencing reality at the beginning of this chapter. After training as a surgeon, this subsequently famous poet apparently never practiced medicine. When he was fourteen, his mother died of tuberculosis. His brother had TB as well. Caring for this brother, the poet also contracted tuberculosis and eventually succumbed to it. John Keats was only 25 years old.

People have known about tuberculosis for around 20,000 years. Like syphilis, it will likely never go away. Today we know that TB is closely related to HIV. In addition, it is causing problems due to its resistance to multiple drug regimens.

I wonder how many cases I may have misdiagnosed in my more than four decades of medical practice. The admonition of Hippocrates to "do no harm" lingers in the mind of every physician, including, I am sure, those who cared for Eleanor Roosevelt.

Obviously, diagnosing tuberculosis and treating patients with this disease was time consuming. Running behind again seemed to be the norm in my time management. However, helping patients with facing realities of an age-old disease also helped *me* to better face life and its realities.

Chapter 8

The Tobacco Holocaust: A Call to Action

"Cigarette smoking is clearly identified as the chief cause of death in our society."

— C. Everett Koop, M.D.

Mr. Hobart Samuelson was a very bright man. He had Type 2 diabetes along with hypertension. I had seen him in the office for several years. Mr. Samuelson had been a former smoker, as well, and had had a persistent cough. One day he came to the office for symptoms of headache and numbness about his face along with difficulty speaking, in terms of forming words. A chest x-ray was non-revealing for any masses or areas that would be concerning for lung cancer. He had imaging studies of his brain, including an MRI scan. He had numerous areas of obvious metastatic disease throughout his brain. A subsequent CT scan of his chest showed a single, small focus of a speculated (star shaped) mass in the left upper lobe of his lung. With a lung biopsy, he was found to have a particular kind of lung cancer referred to as a small cell type. The pathologist determines the cell type of lung cancer by looking at the tissue with a microscope; he also looks at the genetic biomarkers. Mr. Samuelson underwent chemotherapy for the cancer along with radiation to the brain. Unfortunately, he died in a few months.

About 15% of lung cancer cases are of the small cell type. 85% are non-small cell cancers. The non-small cell cancers include adenocarcinoma, squamous cell carcinomas, and large cell lung carcinoma. Small cell lung cancer (SMLC) is a particularly bad form of cancer – the most aggressive – with a seemingly greater propensity to spread to the brain. It is also the type of lung cancer most strongly associated with cigarette smoking.

Mr. Samuelson is only one of many cases of lung cancer that I have seen through the years. In fact, they are too numerous to remember. Lung cancer is the biggest *cance*r killer in the U.S. today. This includes both men and women. While breast cancer is more *common* in women, more women *die* of lung cancer than breast cancer. In fact, there is a famous linear graph in medical statistics that shows lung cancer deaths overtaking breast cancer deaths as early as 1987. *Overall*, the most common cause of death in the U.S. is coronary artery disease with heart attacks. However, there is a big "However" here. This is just my opinion and not necessarily that of other medical professionals. It has been known for some time that in smokers the number of lung cancer deaths is parallel to the number of deaths from heart attacks. *My own personal opinion is that lung cancer deaths, primarily caused by tobacco use, have overtaken deaths from heart attacks.* My reasoning follows.

When a patient has a heart attack, physicians will list the cause of death on the death certificate as heart disease or coronary artery disease. This is especially true when there is no other obvious cause of death. It is easy to see why the vital statistics are skewed toward declaring heart attacks as the leading cause of death.

However, in the case of lung cancer, physicians do not like to use the word "cancer" unless there is strong evidence for such a diagnosis. If the doctor simply writes "lung cancer" as the cause of death, the State Health Department will return the death certificate to the physician for a more detailed description, including location and cell type of the cancer. A biopsy would have proven the cell type. However, if the patient were unable to undergo a biopsy, there would not be a way to determine the cell type. With this lack of required information for the death certificate, the physician often opts to choose another diagnosis as the cause of death.

As a result, fewer lung cancer deaths are reported. This obviously influences the "vital statistics" in any state in the U.S.

There are approximately 480,000 deaths from tobacco use annually in the U.S. *That is about 1,315 deaths per day.* More people die in the U.S. yearly from tobacco than all of the Americans who died in the four years of World War II (403,000 Americans). C. Everett Koop, the famous Surgeon General in President Ronald Reagan's administration, stated, "By the year 2050, 500 million people will die from smoking. Now, that is a Vietnam War every day for 27 years. That's the Titanic sinking every 27 minutes for 27 years." Most of these deaths are from lung cancer and emphysema (COPD).

As mentioned previously, heart disease is the number one cause of death in the United States, with cancer as number two. There is debate about the third leading cause of death – emphysema or medical mistakes. In fact, heart disease, lung cancer, and emphysema are all associated with smoking and spitting tobacco. (Chewing tobacco is too "nice" a term to use.) Smoking is also associated with hardening of the arteries, including peripheral vascular disease (PVD) which is hardening of the arteries in the legs, causing calf and thigh claudication (pain in the affected muscle with exercise such as walking up a hill). Smoking is also a large risk factor in stroke, heart attack, pancreatic cancer, cancer of the cervix, or birth canal, cancer of the esophagus, bladder cancer, and cancer of the larynx, or voice box. In fact, tobacco use is a near 100% risk factor for cancer of the larynx.

The statistics for the world population and their tobacco use are even more staggering. For comparison purposes, I will use diseases not often associated with our local community, yet are major killers.

The following diseases take a great toll on the life of the world's population. Annually, malaria kills about 600,000 to 800,000 people. Tuberculosis kills about 2,000,000, while HIV and AIDS kill 3,000,000. All told, that is 5,600,000 to 5,800,000 people who die annually from these three diseases. On the other hand, tobacco kills more people in the world every year than all three of these horrid diseases combined – more than 6,000,000 deaths per year.

What about the opioid crisis? This is clearly a major health problem. In Tennessee, in 2017, there were about 1,300 opioid overdose deaths. This rate is higher statistically than the national rate, yet in the same year, over 11,400 people were reported to have died in our state from diseases associated with tobacco use. (Remember my opinion stated earlier about death statistics and tobacco-related diseases.) In 2015, about 32% of Tennessee high school youth reported using some type of tobacco product.

American tobacco companies are the main source of the tobacco problem in our country and, indeed, in the world. The main customer of American tobacco companies are children and youth, including high school and college-aged people. 90% of all new tobacco customers come from these ages. Only 10% or less of their new customers are adults.

About 35 years ago, I was seeing Mrs. Georgia Turnbull in the hospital. A former smoker, she was dying of lung cancer. On medications for pain, she suddenly sat up in the hospital bed one day and gave a tearful command, "Dr. Reed, please make me die." Witnessing her terrible suffering, I could no longer be complacent about the tobacco holocaust.

I had an opportunity to join a community group to improve the healthcare of the good people of Kingsport and Sullivan County, Tennessee. With the help of many other professionals and local citizens, we formed the Nicotine-free ME organization. ME stands for Mountain Empire, a name given our region of the country. We have been involved in education about the harmful effects of tobacco with our own local children and youth. Our group talks with several hundred children each year. We heavily emphasize the main reasons why children and youth start using tobacco products. Peer pressure is the number one reason. Feeling older and more mature is an important cause. Parents and siblings who use tobacco products definitely influence the children to use the products despite the bad smell associated with tobacco. Advertising also continues to be a major factor. American tobacco companies prey on our children and youth with regard to all these factors. They emphasize youthfulness, healthiness, sexuality, dealing with life stresses, and sports. There has been evidence of American tobacco companies giving away free cigarettes and spitting tobacco products to children in less developed countries. These companies have hit China, with its 1.3 billion population, hard. In fact, about one million people die in China yearly from smoking – from emphysema and lung cancer.

Today, American tobacco companies are investing in the nation's new pastime – vaping, or electronic smoking. The reason is simple. They are investing in companies to entice youth to start using nicotine-containing products. Nicotine addiction is the direct route to cigarette use. Nicotine is more addicting than alcohol and as addicting as heroin. Nicotine is the ammunition of American tobacco companies that is used in their warfare against the health of Americans. All of this is done in the name of profit. Someone once said, "In fact, tobacco is the only product sold in the entire world that, if used exactly according to the manufacturers' suggestions, is 100% guaranteed to cause harm to your health."

The year 2020 marks my thirty years in youth tobacco prevention. I present a series of slides to fifth and sixth graders at various city and county schools. These presentations discuss the harmful effects of smoking and spitting tobacco use. However, the main event in our presentation is the testimony of patients and local citizens who volunteer their time to talk about how tobacco has affected their lives and the lives of their families. The stories are often quite sad and enlist tears from children and teachers alike. One patient who lost his voice box to tobacco is unable to speak, so he communicates by writing answers to questions on his whiteboard. Without spoken word, his message is always loud and clear. I have always been intrigued by the children's questions for these speakers, considering they are only ten to twelve years old. The most fascinating question was one asked in January 2019 from a little unnamed boy who asked the patient without a voice box, "From where do you get your courage to come and speak to us kids?" I almost fainted at the maturity of this young man's question. His teachers were amazed as well. His question was very meaningful to me. It does take tremendous courage to stand up in front of people and relate your mistakes in life in order to help other people. I only wish I had the courage of these patients and friends!

Additional benefits come as a result of our visiting these schools. The patients, most of whom have experienced the diseases associated with smoking, develop a feeling of self-worth. They are doing something to help their fellow man. Sadly, though, most eventually die from these diseases earlier than otherwise expected. We still have one patient who speaks to the children via a video on my Power Point presentation. He has been dead over fourteen years, but his message continues to live on.

These patients and I have devoted countless hours in our quest to teach the harmful effects of tobacco. We stand strong in our commitment! They take time out of their days to spend with the children. I have done these presentations on my day off, or my "golf day" as I call it (I don't play golf!), or rearranged my schedule of patients to accommodate the schools. Although my retinue and I have not employed any scientific measurement process to gauge our success, we nevertheless continue forward. At least we have always been confident that our efforts would not "go up in smoke." Teaching children about the harmful effects of tobacco is tantamount to the adage that "An ounce of prevention is worth a pound of cure."

Running behind had now become a proud trademark of my determination to curb the tobacco holocaust. When a patient would occasionally frown about my tardiness caused by visiting a school, I would try not to feel guilty but would think to myself that one of the definitions of the word "doctor" is "teacher". Teaching children about America's number one drug problem has been my proudest accomplishment in practicing preventive medicine.

Chapter 9

The "Oh, by the Way" Diagnoses

"Wherever the art of medicine is loved, there is also love of humanity."

— Hippocrates

Early on in my U. S. Navy service, I decided to do an internal medicine residency when my Navy service ended, knowing that it would provide a solid, thorough knowledge of medicine that would allow me to be the best *diagnostician* I could be. As a result, I would also be able to *treat* patients' problems in the best way possible.

One thing I have learned through the years about quality medical treatment is that the kind of care a patient receives is more dependent on the person delivering the care than the particular specialty that they practice. A prestigious doctor who is chairman of an internal medicine department at a top medical center may see the patient who gets a diagnosis and good treatment. In actuality, the patient may actually have received better care from a small town doctor who likes people, spends time with them, enjoys making correct diagnoses, and employs careful, skillful judgement in providing the best overall treatment. It was actually a family practice resident who discovered a heart murmur in my son when he was first admitted to the hospital, helping to establish a diagnosis of endocarditis. (See Chapter 7.) The cognitive skills of the local doctor may actually be better than someone in academia. For example, depending on his education, training, and experience, a good family practitioner may actually make a diagnosis that no one else has been able to make. Dr. Jerome Groopman makes this point in his book, "How Doctors Think," a must read for all medical providers and patients alike.

Near the beginning of my career, I started keeping an index card in my shirt pocket, a routine that served me well through all my years of my medical training and practice. The card provided a convenient place to keep notes about unusual symptoms, signs, or abnormal laboratory results and would encourage me to review these details at the end of the day or in the evening. Often the list would be somewhat lengthy, in which case the card would stay with me for more than one day. In addition, there were times when my diagnostic acumen would limit me. A patient may have had a symptom which left me clueless as to its cause. The question was then listed on my index card and not discarded until the question was answered. After my service in the Navy, I started my residency training in internal medicine, or "medicine" as Dr. Gene Stollerman called it. Internal medicine is about treating the whole patient, including details that others might overlook. In fact, the process through which an internist diagnoses and treats diseases of the adult patient can make him or her seem like a medical detective. The very name "internal medicine" itself refers to getting to the internal part of the patient's possibly elusive problem and not to the physical internal organs. Becoming proficient in the "basics" of medicine, as Dr. Stollerman wanted us to, allowed us to have the tools necessary to uncover the mysteries of the patients' problems. Acting as a medical detective, the internist gets to the heart of the mystery by using these tools to obtain a good history and physical examination of the patient. This allows the doctor to delve into the depths of the patient's problems. As a result, the right diagnosis can be made.

The clinician must often ask the same question in multiple ways in an effort to find the words or terms that finally click for the patient, allowing them to understand what the clinician is asking and then giving the information being sought. Of course, the doctor only does this after carefully listening to the patient first. My internal medicine training taught me to do this, and it usually works. For example, during the history, I would ask a patient who was complaining of chest symptoms if they had actually experienced any "chest discomfort." If the patient did not know what the symptoms of chest discomfort were, I would try to find a different word or question or give more detail to get the needed information. I might ask if they had exertional chest symptoms such as squeezing or tightening or pressure in their chest -symptoms of angina which was brought on by exertion, physical activity, or emotions and was relieved by rest. Since women often describe a sensation of shortness of breath when experiencing angina, I would be sure to ask them about that particular symptom. Spending time to get answers to these questions is important since angina (heart pain) is simply a historical finding with no particular EKG finding, lab test, or imaging study to define it. Positive answers to the various questions asked during the history can lead the physician to undertake further testing such as stress testing to look for evidence of coronary artery disease (blockages in the coronary arteries that can lead to heart attack and sudden death). The symptom of angina is very important since it is one of the ways that coronary artery disease, the major cause of death in the U.S., manifests itself. Therefore, asking questions in different ways is a good tactic to use to be certain that the correct diagnosis is made.

I remember the day when Mr. George Ackerman came to my office for his very first visit. In his 60's, he had retired from the laundry business. He had a history of poorly controlled diabetes, high blood pressure, high cholesterol, and had previously been a smoker. He had many risk factors for angina and coronary artery disease.

Based on his risk factors, I asked questions carefully to see if he had any symptoms of angina. He seemed to have none of the usual symptoms. After spending approximately sixty minutes doing the history and physical examination, I stood up to tell him that I had enjoyed meeting him and would be in contact with him after reviewing his labs from that morning. As I opened the door to leave, he stopped me with a concerned look on his face. He said, "Oh, by the way, Doc, I forgot to tell you something." I sat back down and quietly listened as he spontaneously shared additional history. He said that his mailbox was at the bottom of a long, steep driveway. While ordinary activity around his house, such as yard work, did not elicit chest discomfort or chest pain, walking back up that drive way had been associated with a tight sensation in his chest and neck as well as nausea and a sense of breathlessness. These symptoms may have been exacerbated by potential bad news about his family that he anticipated in the mail any day.

Mr. Ackerman eventually underwent stress testing that was abnormal and led to a coronary artery catheterization. Coronary artery catheterization is done by placing a tube in the groin or wrist that is then threaded into the arteries of the heart to define stenosis, or blockages that might be amenable to stenting during the procedure. Because all of his arteries were badly diseased with multiple blockages, stenting was not an option. After having multi-vessel coronary artery bypass grafting (CABG), he has continued to do well through the years. Unfortunately, after the CABG procedure was done, he developed other areas of blockages in the carotid arteries (arteries in the front of the neck that take oxygenated blood to the brain). This required subsequent stenting. In addition, he developed kidney disease related to poor control of his diabetes.

Another patient who surprised me with "Oh, by the way" physical findings was Mr. Herman Donelson. When Mr. Donelson first came to my office, no particular problem was found on examination of his abdomen. Toward the end of the examination, I left the room for a moment. Upon re-entering the room, I happened to notice a movement in his abdomen. Repeat, careful evaluation revealed a large abdominal aortic aneurysm. He was referred for an open repair procedure and did well through the years.

Helen Donelson, Herman's wife, had seen me in the office the prior week. One morning she fell and injured her chest and later felt a lump in her breast. Late in the day, she came by the office. Finding the front door locked, she came around the back of the building and pecked on the window. She was brought in through the side door. With a nurse in the room, I examined her and found an obvious bruise and hematoma (pump knot) in the affected breast, but no serious disease was found. She was obviously very grateful.

I never knew what surprises the "Oh, by the way" symptoms or physical findings might reveal. Comments that the patient made going out the door could sometimes point to serious disease. As it turned out, I came to appreciate this unexpected way of making an unexpected diagnosis. It has mainly to do with listening, a vitally important part of the *art* of medicine. Mr. Ackerman, Mr. and Mrs. Donelson, and many other such patients caused me to run behind each day. I learned, however, that these "Oh, by the way" complaints and physical findings, which took extra time, often led to significant discoveries. Keeping ahead of the patients' problems, but running behind in time was often not only necessary, but could be lifesaving.

Chapter 10

The Patient and His Bull

"There are no traffic jams along the extra mile."

— Roger Staubach

Ronald Harris was a very nice man who smoked constantly. He had diabetes that was always poorly controlled. I routinely checked his A1Cs. A1C is the most popular method of determining control of diabetes. It gives us an idea of the average blood sugar over eight to ten weeks with a normal value being less than 6.5. Depending on the patient's age and overall health, an A1C around 7.0 correlates with good control of the blood sugar in someone with Type 2 diabetes,

Mr. Harris' A1Cs were always in the range of 10-13. Continuous smoking, poor blood pressure control, and hyperlipidemia (high cholesterol, or fats, in the blood) accompanied his poor diabetes control. Since he struggled financially, taking insulin in proper doses was problematic due to its high cost. Mr. Harris also had heart and kidney disease. His wife was in poor health as well.

He lived on a small farm in Carter County where his family owned cattle, including a 1600-pound bull named Gilbert. When bills accumulated, including medical bills, he needed more money. Thus, he decided to sell Gilbert.

One of my favorite past-times is to visit local cattle auctions. I enjoy seeing the cattle and observing the interaction of the buyers and sellers with the auctioneer's voice giving a lively, festive tone to the whole event. One day at a cattle sale, I noticed Mr. Harris was there, too. After coming over to sit next to me, he began telling me why he was there to sell Gilbert. He also shared with me about his wife's worsening health. As a result, his increasing financial problems led to his being at the cattle sale. He was hoping to get as much money as he could from selling their bull.

As it turns out, I had come to know one of the buyers from a slaughterhouse. Mr. Reece was known for "adjusting" his bid price up for people he knew well. Mr. Harris was unaware of these types of financial dealings, so with his permission I talked with Mr. Reece about his financial situation. He said he would help Mr. Harris out. That particular day bulls were bringing only about $.65 - $.68 per pound. When Gilbert came into the ring for sale, the bidding was low. Mr. Reece stepped up and bid $0.76 per pound for the bull. As a result, Mr. Harris took a bigger check home that day. Although the difference in the amount of money was not huge, my patient thanked me.

I actually had a motive for doing this for my patient. The motive was the hope that my rapport with him would improve and therefore would motivate him to keep his diabetes and other medical problems under better control. While the intended effects of my actions did not materialize, I knew I had done the best I could for him in and out of the office.

Continuing to smoke, he remained oblivious to his cardiovascular risk status. Diabetes does not usually *hurt* until there is sufficient vascular damage to interfere with vision, kidney function, or nerve function in the legs. Blindness and dialysis following kidney failure often become synonymous with years of poorly controlled diabetes. Nerve damage can result in numbness and neuropathic ulcers in the feet (peripheral neuropathy). As with the general population, most often the cause of death is cardiovascular with heart attack as the number one cause of death for these patients.

I spent a lot of time in office visits and phones calls with Mr. Harris. It made me run behind with my remaining patients. In this case, though, I felt pretty good about running behind. And that's no bull!

Chapter 11

The Missing Narratives: Cases of Poisoning

"Pretending must never be a part of doctoring. The physician who listens to a patient describe his or her symptoms but hears no clues to the presence of disease is pretending."

— "Essays from the Heart"
by J. Willis Hurst, M.D.

In my first year of internal medicine residency at the University of Tennessee in Memphis, I was in charge of four medical students and two interns. One day we admitted a patient who was unconscious, was bleeding from the rectum, and had a very low blood pressure. His name was Jacob Whitehead. At his admission, we did not know that he had taken a large dose of arsenic in a suicide attempt. Once we became aware of this hours after his admission, we began treating him for the arsenic poisoning. Because of our inability to keep his blood pressure up adequately, however, we were unable to save his life. Part of the problem with our treatment of Mr. Whitehead was the lack of narrative. He was unconscious, and initially there was no family around to give us his medical history or any clues about his ingestion of the poison. This narrative would have changed the focus of our treatment and possibly saved his life.

During the treatment of Mr. Whitehead's arsenic ingestion, I learned a great deal about this type of poisoning. I felt that the next time I saw a case of acute arsenic poisoning my "tool kit" would be full. As it turns out, after four and a half years of post-graduate training and over 40 years of medical practice, I never saw another case of acute arsenic poisoning. However, unknown to me at the time, I would later encounter arsenic poisoning in a different manner.

After my residency, I did a general internal medicine fellowship at the University of Tennessee during which I worked with a very experienced physician, Dr. Gerald Plitman, for eighteen months. My one-on-one time with him provided me with a wonderful learning experience. He received a lot of referrals from doctors in Mississippi and Arkansas. One of these patients was Oliver Silverman from Clarksdale, Mississippi. He had presented with anemia, or low blood count. The cause of this had been elusive. Dr. Plitman always said that 70-80% of cases of anemia could be diagnosed from the history (the narrative) and physical examination along with the examination of the blood smear. This involves looking at the cellular components of blood, including the eight-micron biconcave disc form of the red blood cells. In my mind, Dr. Plitman was always correct in his diagnoses. He was an outstanding clinician!

I was elated that Dr. Plitman had asked me to see Mr. Silverman who had anemia. On examination of the blood smear, he had "basophilic stippling." This condition describes the appearance of "granules" in red blood cells and has been found to be RNA. It represents a disturbance in erythropoiesis (the genesis, or making of red blood cells in the bone marrow) and may be found in many different conditions affecting the bone marrow. Basophilic stippling may be characteristic of, but not diagnostic of, heavy metal poisoning. Heavy metals to which people may be exposed can include arsenic, lead, and mercury.

Besides anemia, he had evidence of dementia. His wife, who seemed attentive, had been aware of his cognitive impairment for a few years.

Interestingly, he also had a wrist drop, a condition in which the patient has difficulty raising his wrist above the horizontal plane.

So, we had a patient with a triad of signs - anemia, dementia, and a wrist drop. One etiologic factor that can cause this triad of signs is heavy metal poisoning. There was clearly no history of any such exposure, including any occupational exposure. Along with other laboratory tests, a urine test was ordered. The arsenic level in the urine was in the 100,000 ranges, an extraordinarily high level. Dr. Plitman discharged Mr. Silverman and contacted his doctor in Clarksdale for follow up. He had likely been exposed to arsenic for years. While someone may have poisoned him, I never heard the details of further investigations since my fellowship ended, and I moved to my own practice elsewhere.

Later in my career, I met Mr. Jerome Masters. He had come to the hospital for throat pain. He was admitted for an underlying metabolic acidosis of unknown origin. Metabolic acidosis is a serious condition in which acid builds up in the blood; it may portend a poor outcome for the patient. He had no kidney function impairment or evidence of sepsis (infection in the blood) initially. During the ensuing days, his metabolic acidosis worsened. He then developed acute renal (kidney) failure. The nephrologist (kidney specialist) saw him in consultation. With his many years of experience, he simply asked the patient what substance he had ingested. The patient responded that he had drunk a large glass of antifreeze in a suicide attempt. I had not thought about asking this direct question! Despite days of therapy, the patient died. He refused dialysis. Upon looking back over this case after the patient died, I discovered two overlooked clues in his presentation. Obviously, if the patient had told us that he drank antifreeze, perhaps early life saving dialysis could have been instituted.

One clue was the complaint of throat pain. However, many diagnoses can cause this malady. The other clue was his initial urine analysis. Review showed that his urine was full of calcium oxalate crystals. Calcium oxalate crystals in the urine are generally only clinically significant when they form kidney stones. However, ethylene glycol (antifreeze) ingestion can *cause* the calcium oxalate crystals to form in the urine and therefore be a clue to such poisoning. Formation of these crystals can also be caused by other factors, including eating a large amount of rhubarb.

William Osler, the father of America medicine, said, "Listen to the patient, he will tell you his diagnosis." I have always believed this adage, so I listen as carefully as I can to the patient's narrative. The patient will not tell you the exact medical diagnosis but will often give enough historical clues and have subtle physical and laboratory abnormalities that point the clinician in the right direction. However, in two of these cases, the clues were quite elusive. I am glad that, at least with this patient, I cannot be accused of "pretending" to listen.

Although two of the patients died, I did not attribute their deaths directly to my lack of time or the amount of thought I put into their diagnosis and treatment. The practice of medicine can be compared to the game of baseball. Every time you are at bat, you would like to hit a home run but, in the end, all you ever remember are the strikeouts.

These patients required an enormous amount of time. I have always tried to work hard for my patients. Recently a patient told me that he appreciated my having taken good care of his mother who, by the way, lived to be 100. I had seen her in the ER years ago for a hospital admission. He said that after examining her, I left her bedside for about thirty minutes. He then found me in an office looking through his mother's records. He was very appreciative of my effort and time spent. Later, he said that my efforts "just go to prove that a person can work hard and do a good job without necessarily being brilliant." I just smiled and thanked him.

This time, running behind did not result in medical success as defined by simply living longer. In medical practice, however, I believe we are called to be faithful always and successful when possible. Hippocrates once said, "Cure sometimes, treat often, and comfort always." Running behind was worth the effort in these cases.

Chapter 12

An Unusual Case of Leg Pain

"He who knows syphilis knows medicine."

— Sir William Osler

After volunteering for the U.S. Navy in 1975, I was stationed at China Lake Naval Weapons Center in China Lake, California from 1976 until early 1978. I worked in the base's Dispensary as a GMO, or general medical officer, seeing active duty personnel and retired sailors and their families.

One such patient was Jean Cortez. She was the widow of a former Navy Chief who lived in the local town of Ridgecrest. She had come to my care complaining of leg pain. She described her leg pain as severe, relentless, and unassociated with back pain or any history of falls or trauma. The pain seemed to be lacinating, or lightning type pain. She also had some subjective and objective signs of leg weakness. In addition, she had diminished reflexes in the affected lower extremity.

There is an old saying in internal medicine, "People with unusual symptoms generally have uncommon symptoms of a common disease rather than common symptoms of an uncommon disease." However, this patient seemed to be an exception to this rule

Routine studies and lumbar spine x-rays failed to disclose the exact nature of her malady. Use of CT scans was just beginning but we did not have one at our facility. MRI scanning was not known in those days.

An additional point should be made here. I reviewed her x-rays *myself* before sending them to a radiologist at the Long Beach Naval Hospital in Long Beach, California. The radiologist subsequently sent me a written report of his findings. Throughout my career, when I ordered an x-ray or other imaging procedures, I generally reviewed them myself either before or after the radiologist sent their written report. Today, digitalization of imaging procedures makes this review easier. As an example, if a patient is diagnosed with pneumonia, the physician ordering the x-ray must review the actual chest x-ray. Then, the patient and the patient's area of pneumonia become firmly entrenched in the doctor's brain. (A picture is worth a thousand words.) *In my opinion, not reviewing an imaging procedure is tantamount to a mechanic reviewing a potential mechanical problem with a vehicle without ever actually seeing that vehicle.* I cannot overemphasize this point enough! Incidentally, the same can be said about reviewing abnormalities found on mammograms, CAT scans, and MRI scans. In addition, I have found a real advantage in reviewing the imaging procedures with a different radiologist than the one who made the original reading. In this way, the primary physician gets a "second opinion" about the reading of that procedure. I have found this to be particularly helpful over the last forty years.

Mrs. Cortez's history indicated that she had had more than *one* husband in the past and had lived in many areas of the world. She denied any illicit relationships in the past. Additional laboratory studies confirmed a positive VDRL, a test for syphilis. Neurosyphilis, a late complication of syphilis, seemed to be a potential diagnosis, so a lumbar puncture, or spinal tap, was done to examine her spinal fluid. The VDRL test on her spinal fluid, as well as subsequent testing, confirmed that she had complications of syphilis with neurosyphilis. Specifically, her diagnosis was tabes dorsalis. She received intravenous penicillin and made a good response.

I had seen cases of presumed neurosyphilis presenting in late stages as dementia and had also seen cardiovascular complications with aortic syphilis with aortic insufficiency (leakage of the aortic valve.) The syphilis organism, called a spirochete, infects the aorta in this disease.

This, however, was the first case of neurosyphilis with tabes doralis that I had seen.

One further point is to be made here. When seeing a patient with unusual symptoms and signs, doing a sedimentation rate, or simply sed rate, is a common practice that the physician may consider. The sed rate is a blood test which measures the rate at which red blood cells settle over a period of sixty minutes. It is a very sensitive but very nonspecific test for inflammation. Perhaps a better admonition for doctors today, however, is that, "When considering doing a sed rate in patients with unusual symptoms and signs, the patient may not need a sed rate but needs a *doctor*." In other words, seeing a patient with unusual symptoms and signs means that the doctor goes back to the drawing board, so to speak --- goes back to the history and physical examination and starts again.

By the way, I ordered a sed rate on Mrs. Cortez. It was normal. Therefore, I had to go back to the drawing board.

As mentioned previously, my mentor, Dr. Gene Stollerman, said, "The most important thing we can give a patient is the proper diagnosis." This patient took a lot of extra time to diagnose and treat. Fifteen minutes spent with her would have yielded no diagnosis and no proper treatment.

Tabes dorsalis is a complicated and elusive diagnosis. Sir Arthur Conan Doyle, author of 'Stories of Sherlock Holmes," did postgraduate work on tabes dorsalis to obtain his M.D. degree in 1885.

Obviously, once again, with this patient, I was running behind. Medical literature was reviewed and infectious disease physicians were consulted at the San Diego Naval Hospital in San Diego, California. The review and the consultations took a lot of time. My only hope was that with my next patient I could be as thoughtful and scientific with their diagnosis. Good patient care always demands such diligence.

Chapter 13

Diagnostic and Therapeutic Dilemmas

"I have learned since to be a better student and to be ready to say to my fellow students, 'I do not know.'"

— Sir William Osler

Many patients have symptoms and signs that are elusive. Symptoms are findings discovered from discussion with the patient, called the history, while signs are findings from the physical examination. In general, the probability of getting the right diagnosis is greater when a greater amount of TIME is spent with the patient. In addition, making an actual list of their complaints and findings for additional study in the off-hours can be very helpful as well. Keeping this kind of notes was the purpose for my always having an index card in my white coat pocket.

I have been to many conferences during my career as an internist. Oftentimes, unusual cases are presented during these conferences. Doctors in the audience are asked to find the correct diagnosis for these cases. I have always been impressed by how many well-trained and experienced physicians, including myself, have a hard time getting the right diagnosis. Many times, I have wondered why patients in our own practices who present with diagnostic dilemmas could not undergo this same scrutiny at a meeting of local physicians, or at least at a meeting of the same specialty colleagues. In other words, a team of physicians could discuss that patient's problems and perhaps reach a diagnosis as a result of the collaboration. After all, the team approach is used in large academic medical centers and other disciplines such as in engineering. Certainly, referrals or consultations are the more common mode of teamwork in medicine. However, it would clearly be better to have a face-to-face encounter with colleagues.

When I was in the Navy, I saw Commander Joseph Haysworth. He had retired, having previously served as the Executive Officer on a US Navy cruiser. He had been having fever for several months. As it turned out, he had previously had multiple evaluations, including an examination at the prestigious Johns Hopkins Hospital in Baltimore. Nevertheless, I did a thorough history and physical examination. There was no particular epidemiologic clue as to any possible infectious cause of his fever. Fever has always been a favorite symptom of mine in medicine to evaluate. I consider myself very fortunate to have heard the great Louis Weinstein, M.D. discuss this topic at Harvard. He had written the famous landmark article entitled "Fever of Unknown Origin" which was printed in the prestigious *New England Journal of Medicine* in 1950.

Like his previous physicians and after discussion and evaluations, I, too, was unable to find a cause for Commander Haysworth's fever. How helpful it would have been if there had been a roundtable of physicians to discuss his findings!

Mrs. Gladys Hightower was in her early fifties when I first saw her. She was having high fevers and joint pain, and had a rash on her arms and legs. Her symptoms and signs, as well as her laboratory findings, were not consistent with any infectious disease, including any tick-borne disease, such as Rocky Mountain Spotted fever. Her pattern of fever, joint pain, and the absence of other findings pointed to a diagnosis of Adult Still's disease, also known as juvenile rheumatoid arthritis beginning in adulthood. Her fever eventually subsided, and she did well with NSAIDS, or non-steroidal anti-inflammatory drugs such as Ibuprofen. Eventually she was referred to a rheumatologist. However, it would have been so enlightening to have been able to meet in the same room with multiple colleagues and discuss her case.

Another interesting patient was Mrs. Caroline Purkey from Kingsport, Tennessee. An elderly woman, Mrs. Purkey had underlying kidney disease, anemia, and high blood pressure. She had come to see me for a complaint of shortness of breath. Careful examination revealed that she had a heart murmur. The murmur seemed to be consistent with mitral stenosis. Mitral stenosis is rarely seen these days. It is a condition caused by scarring on the mitral valve (the heart valve between the left atrium and left ventricle). The scarring that occurs on the valve results in a constricted valve opening. The most common cause of this condition is inflammation from acute rheumatic fever, which is seen less often today. The resultant murmur produces a diastolic murmur. This type of murmur occurs during diastole, the phase when the left ventricle is at rest and not pumping. The murmur has a particular sound and is described as "the sound of an oxcart slowly crossing a wooden bridge in the distance." The murmur also occurs after an OS, or opening snap, which is produced by the opening of the diseased or thickened valve leaflets. An echocardiogram was done that seemingly showed only mild mitral stenosis. I discussed her case with the cardiologist. He did not feel that further evaluation was needed. She died in a few months from multisystem disease. I still believe today that her underlying problem was indeed mitral stenosis. On hindsight, it would have been much better to discuss her findings with a group of physicians, including multiple cardiologists.

Mrs. Deloris Agee from Elizabethton, Tennessee had been in the hospital for treatment of dehydration. Despite I.V. fluids, her creatinine, an indirect measure of kidney function, continued to rise. Unfortunately, no one had bothered to look carefully at her urine. She was subsequently found to have red cell casts and a lot of protein in the urine. Excessive protein in the urine is indicative of a leaking glomerulus (the filtering unit of the kidney). In other words, excessive protein is indicative of serious kidney disease. Red cell casts indicate acute nephritis (active inflammation in the kidney). The red cell casts and increased protein were consistent with acute glomerulonephritis. These findings and the symptoms of joint pain, along with certain blood tests, pointed to possible SLE (systemic lupus erythematosus, or, simply, lupus). Having trained at the University of Tennessee in Memphis helped me to make the diagnosis since we saw many cases of lupus there. Mrs. Agee was referred to a rheumatologist and nephrologist for treatment. She has done well to this date! During the time of her evaluation, I longed for a face-to-face round table conference to discuss her problems, rather than just phone calls.

Lupus is a disease that can be elusive to diagnose. Although I did not see the patient, I knew of a young girl who had pain in her heel. Heel pain is usually a localized condition such as tendonitis. Apparently, no further evaluation was done to look for evidence of a systemic disease. As it turns out, she developed acute kidney failure from glomerulonephritis (kidney inflammation) that stemmed from a vasculitis (inflammation of the blood vessels). She died within six months of fulminant kidney failure. Perhaps if a urine analysis had been done early on, her life might have been saved! This is especially true if her urine had shown evidence of red cell casts and protein. As it turns out, her heel pain was likely an enthesitis associated with the vasculitis. An enthesitis is an inflammation at the site of the attachment of a tendon to a bone. Her underlying diagnosis was possibly lupus.

Therapeutic dilemmas occur as well. Mr. Jimmy Greene was from St Clair, Tennessee. He was 32 years old and had come to the office for a complaint of chest discomfort. He had felt tightness, or pressure, in his chest while running the bases playing softball. A clinical diagnosis of angina pectoris, or heart pain, was made. On the treadmill, he had severe changes indicative of multi-vessel coronary artery disease. He then underwent a heart catheterization. During catheterization, a tube is placed in the femoral artery in the groin and eventually into the heart in order to place x-ray contrast dye so that any blockages in the coronary arteries can be seen. The coronary arteries supply the heart muscle with oxygenated blood. Mr. Greene's coronary arteries were found to be small and filled with multiple blockages.

Local cardiovascular surgeons felt that he was not a good surgical candidate because of his severe disease and small coronary arteries. He was then referred to a large hospital in Nashville, Tennessee where the surgeons also agreed that he was a poor surgical candidate. The patient was subsequently referred to the world-famous Mayo Clinic in Rochester, Minnesota. The chief of cardiology agreed with the other surgeons. However, the Mayo Clinic cardiologists then *held a round table discussion with their fellow cardiologists.* Their decision was to repeat the treadmill test and discuss his case again. His treadmill test was repeated and again found to be indicative of severe problems.

Despite the high risk, the cardiologists decided they needed to proceed with surgery. Mr. Greene underwent coronary artery bypass grafting (CABG), did well after surgery, and was discharged after a few days. While he did well at home for a while, he continued to smoke cigarettes and eventually died of a stroke before his fortieth birthday. This case represents the power of physician interactions with multiple consultants for a good honest and open discussion and communication!

Although round table discussions were not possible in our practice setting, I nevertheless often sought consultations with other colleagues and consultants. Medicine is complicated. Making a correct and expedient diagnosis is tantamount to providing excellent patient care!

Sometimes even the most experienced physician cannot come up with a diagnosis using the signs and symptoms with which patients present. This may be because of the rarity of the disease which can make a diagnosis even more elusive. Sometimes internists are criticized for looking for rare diseases in their patients. However, in the aggregate, rare diseases are actually common. In other words, if circulatory disease were to occupy a large circle, infectious diseases another circle, and rheumatic diseases yet another circle, the rare diseases as a whole would occupy a large circle, as well. This is why training in internal medicine in a large university medical center is so important. The internal medicine resident should have exposure to multiple specialties in a referral center to see a large number of patients with many different disease states. A physician has a hard time making the diagnosis of a disease he or she has never seen, let alone never heard of.

These cases of diagnostic and therapeutic dilemmas demand thorough patient conversations and examinations, extra thought, and consultations with other physicians. That adds up to a lot of extra time. Spending time in face-face round table discussions with other physicians would take time, too, but would be of much benefit to patient outcomes. The practitioner involved in such cases will always run behind. However, I can say with certainty that making the correct diagnosis and obtaining the right treatment is always more important than sticking to a schedule

Chapter 14

Dementia, the Sad Diagnosis

There are only four kinds of people in the world: those who have been caregivers, those who are currently caregivers, those who will be caregivers, and those who will need caregivers.

— Rosalyn Carter

Dementia patients are perhaps the saddest cases that a physician can encounter. It robs patients of any meaningful life. This can stretch into years when they have few or no physical problems. I had one patient with Alzheimer's disease who lived for eighteen years. Her husband fed her three times a day – taking around an hour with each meal. When he developed cancer and could no longer care for her, she died within about three weeks. I always tried to be sure of any diagnosis, including ones of dementia. A careful examination must be done each time this diagnosis is suspected. There are so many causes of dementia, including Alzheimer's disease, Lewy body disease often associated with Parkinsonian features, and Pick's disease. Patients with vascular disease may have multiple strokes presenting as dementia. Correctable cases of dementia need to be diagnosed early. These would include pseudo-dementia, or depression, and normal pressure hydrocephalus (NPH). NPH presents with dementia, difficulty with gait called apraxia and urinary difficulties with incontinence.

While NPH can be difficult to diagnose, it can be corrected with a shunt to relieve a build-up of spinal fluid in the brain.

The problem with diagnosing dementia arises when trying to determine the exact onset of symptoms. Unless members of the patient's family relate a memory problem, dementia often goes undiagnosed until at least moderate or severe disease is present. Therefore, testing for the disease should be done early on. A simple screening is as easy as the physician checking the patient's *recall* using the mini mental status exam (MMSE) (See Chapter 3). During this exam, the patient is asked to remember three words given by the physician, such as horse, flower, and town, in order to repeat them later to the physician. In five minutes after giving the words, the physician asks the patient to repeat the words. Another of the questions on a typical MMSE (mini mental status exam) is having the patient write a complete sentence. The results are often surprising and even shocking. Patients with severe dementia may not be able to write anything at all. Others may write a few words and then stop altogether.

My patient Mrs. Jane Crawford can illustrate the heartbreak of these cases. Her son had brought her in for evaluation of memory loss. He worked the night shift and had difficulty bringing her to the office. As I examined Mrs. Crawford, her son appeared to be quite frustrated with her memory loss and the seemingly never-ending care that she needed. He looked exhausted. As the MMSE proceeded, I asked her to write a complete sentence. At first, she seemed to be unable to do this simple task at all. Her son shook his head in frustration at having to wait so long for her response. Finally, she wrote a brief sentence. After reading it, I showed it to the frustrated son with tears in my eyes. As he read it, her son cried. The sentence read, "I love my son." Dementia should never be equated with loss of feelings – only of memory and insight.

One humorous event happened with a patient in whom I had some possible suspicion of memory loss. During the course of the examination, I asked Bud Rogers to repeat the proverbial three words of recall. The problem was that I failed to ask him to repeat these three objects within five minutes, as I had told him I would. When he returned to the office four months later, he exclaimed, "horse, flower and town!" as he shook my hand. Needless to say, it was quite embarrassing but certainly reassured me that memory loss was not one of his problems!

Years ago, a patient who seemed to have dementia fooled me. His daughter said that Mr. Jenkins had memory loss. He also urinated in his bathtub at home. This unusual behavior did, in fact, make me suspect there was something wrong. However, his MMSE score was not that bad. In addition, he told me that he read *Time* magazine regularly. I was certainly perplexed. How could he have dementia and yet read this well-known periodical? One day, I asked his daughter to bring a copy of this magazine with her to his appointment. When asked to read the print, he was unable to do so. As it turns out, he had merely been looking at the pictures. This example demonstrates why the physician must examine the patient in the context of the patient's total social and psychological milieu, in addition to a thorough history and physical examination.

Some of my younger patients had dementia as well. One particular man was Mr. Harvey Burchell. He was in his early fifties. He had presented with symptoms of memory loss and Parkinson's disease while still working for the county. Neurology consultation confirmed that he had a fairly common form of dementia called Lewy body disease. His wife cared for him in the home for many years. Mr. Burchell was a patient who turned out to be one of the saddest cases of dementia that I had seen.

Dementia is not only sad; it is very expensive. The lack of planning for their later years by patients and their families is astounding! It is heartbreaking to hear of the struggles that families have with their members who have been diagnosed with dementia. The cost of care only adds to the frustration. In recent years, I have recommended that patients and families prepare for possible home care, assisted living, or nursing home care with long-term care (LTC) policies or with the use of riders on life insurance policies or annuities.

These cases of evaluation of memory loss took a lot of time. Examination of the patient and discussion with the family were quite time consuming. However, even though it made me run behind in the office, my own memory is filled with good stories about patients with whom taking this extra time hopefully made a difference.

Chapter 15

Alcoholism: The Undiagnosed Disease

"I am more afraid of alcohol than of the bullets of the enemy."

— Stonewall Jackson

As stated previously, the best gift of the doctor to his patient is the correct diagnosis. In my career, alcohol abuse and its effects on the mind and body have been difficult to diagnose. Alcohol ingestion often remains in the "shadows" of the social history that doctors do in examining the patients. The exception would be the patient who comes to the hospital intoxicated. The diagnosis of alcohol abuse often goes undetected because it is not considered to be a potential problem. Often alcohol abuse disorder would be discovered in my practice in the following scenarios:

1. The surgeon calls me and says that the patient has a small nodular liver (cirrhosis) at the time of elective gall bladder removal or other abdominal surgery.
2. Abnormal liver tests are found on routine blood testing leading to imaging studies such as ultrasound that reveals evidence of cirrhosis.
3. The physical examination finding of an enlarged liver or liver with a nodule (lump) that had not been previously discovered despite having seen the patient for years.

4. A liver biopsy is done because of abnormal liver blood tests revealing evidence of cirrhosis consistent with years of drinking alcohol.
5. The newspaper report of public drunkenness or a DUI (driving under the influence). On one occasion, an ER doctor wrote on the ER discharge summary that the patient "smelled of alcohol"

All of these scenarios point to the lack of a good history pertaining to alcohol ingestion. Oftentimes, the provider will not ask details for fear of a confrontation. Also, the patient will deny there is a problem; the patient may say, "I'm a social drinker." The amount of alcohol consumed may seem insignificant to the doctor and the patient. In fact, the amount of alcohol consumed may have little relation to *any* alcohol problem.

A more *detailed* inquiry may reveal the following:

1. The husband confides in you that his wife drinks every day to the point of sleeping all the time and avoiding family activities.
2. The patient has previously had abnormal liver tests.
3. The patient has been through alcohol rehabilitation - previously and now reports that he only drinks "socially."
4. The patient was recently diagnosed with an alcohol problem but does not attend AA regularly.
5. The college student drinks alcohol at parties every weekend and gets drunk with friends.
6. The patient becomes intoxicated on the weekends only. Often getting "buzzed" is not associated with being intoxicated.
7. The patient is the "happy drunk" at parties and never misses work because of drinking.
8. The patient had a DUI several years ago.
9. The husband who always drinks alone.
10. The patient with a sleep disorder.
11. The teenager with a change in attitude or motivation.
12. The patient with a family history of alcoholism

I regularly use the mnemonic "CAGE" in the evaluation of the alcohol history. Sample questions that are related to each letter of the is word are:

"C" Have you ever felt the need to Cut back on your alcohol intake?
"A" Have you felt Annoyed by someone discussing your alcohol ingestion with you?
"G" Have you had Guilt feelings about drinking
"E" Have you had a drink early in the morning as an "Eye opener"?

Each positive answer counts for one point, except for "E" which counts for two points. A score of two to three points indicates a high index of suspicion. A score of four is usually diagnostic of an alcohol problem. This is reviewed in detail in the reference Diagnostic Statistical Manual of Mental Disorders. One must remember that CAGE is a screening tool only and does not establish a definitive diagnosis of alcoholism. An important point to be made is that social drinking has no definite bounds in its definition. It usually refers to alcohol consumption of a modest amount at social functions or "wine with dinner," as an example.

I am not making any moral judgements either. Indeed, I believe the physician should always have a nonjudgmental attitude toward patients. This includes nonjudgmental attitudes toward the patient's religion, politics, income, social welfare status, race, sexual orientation, etc.

In addition, the physical effects are often insidious and missed by the clinicians. Even a careful examination of the patient's abdomen may not reveal the enlarged liver or spleen. The spleen often enlarges due to the liver disease. Abnormal liver tests may be intermittent. In fact, the patient may first present with late stage disease when the patient comes in with evidence of liver cancer associated with cirrhosis or when they come in with vomiting of blood (from esophageal varices – dilated veins at the bottom of the esophagus – caused by the liver disease). Likewise, the patient may first present with heart disease with CHF (congestive heart failure), dementia, or neuropathy (damaged nerves in the arms and legs). They may also present with a low platelet count. Platelets are small particles in the blood that make the blood clot. Occult liver disease may subsequently be found with this lab finding.

Winston Churchill, always known for his drinking, once stated, "My rule of life prescribed as an absolutely sacred rite smoking cigars and also the drinking of alcohol before, after, and if need be during all meals and in the intervals between them". My question to his physician Charles McMoran Wilson (Lord Moran) today would be, "Did you do periodic assessments of his liver status?"

Mr. Charles Green was from Scott County, Virginia. He had several medical problems including hypertension, diabetes, obesity, and lumbar disc disease. He had had some intermittent abnormal liver tests for years. I had never directly inquired in detail about his alcohol intake. On one occasion, a liver biopsy was recommended. He was found to have active hepatitis and findings of alcoholic cirrhosis. I felt bad that I had never taken a full history of his alcohol consumption.

Mr. Frank Irvin, from Bristol, Tennessee had multisystem disease including severe rheumatoid arthritis, hypertension, heart disease, and a known history of liver disease presumably from alcohol. One day he came to see me and was quite tearful. He wanted to stop drinking and change his life completely. I applauded him for his courage and called his insurance company to arrange for hospitalization for alcohol rehabilitation. It took about one hour at the end of a long day to accomplish this. He then decided to beat this disease on his own. Despite my telling him that this would be almost impossible to do, he refused the hospitalization. In the following months and years, he attended AA meetings and came back to see me on a regular basis. He refrained from all alcohol ingestion and became one of the greatest successes in alcohol abuse treatment in my career!

I have come to realize that alcoholism can be treated if the patient wants help and stops denying there is a problem. Denial of alcohol abuse is the major obstacle in the initial treatment. Notice I did not say alcoholism could be cured. I learned that rapport with the provider along with regular AA attendance could change a person's life.

In fact, I believe strongly that those patients who have strong faith in their doctor can be treated more successfully for their alcohol abuse. I agree with William Osler (whom I often quote) who said, "Faith in the gods or in the saints cures one, faith in little pills another, hypnotic suggestion a third, faith in a plain common doctor a fourth."

Alcohol abuse often goes unrecognized by the patient, the family, and, unfortunately, by the medical provider. As the famous preacher John Wesley said, "Strong, and more especially spirituous liquors are a certain, though slow, poison." I must make this important point as a doctor as well. While a person does not have to view alcohol in the same way as Stonewall Jackson, the point to be made by me is that the social drinker, the patient with an alcohol abuse disorder, or the person who suffers from alcoholism may have harmful physical effects from the alcohol that remain completely hidden for many years. Thus my belief that alcohol is an insidious problem! I would admonish physicians to be more adept at obtaining a good history of alcohol ingestion and doing a good physical examination looking for complications of alcohol abuse. The patient's life may be saved!

Much extra time was spent with patients who suffered from alcohol abuse. This was especially true of Mr. Irwin. However, as usual, I felt that patient care precluded any concerns about running behind.

Chapter 16

The Missed Diagnoses: Lessons in Humility

"It is astonishing with how little reading a doctor can practice medicine but it is not astonishing how badly he may do it."

— Sir William Osler

William Osler had a great influence on the practice of modern medicine. Emphasizing the science of medicine was paramount in his teaching physicians in their post-graduate education. He saw the hospital bed as a college classroom. He, in fact, moved the teaching of medicine from the lecture hall to the bedside. He emphasized reading and learning. When I was in training years ago, I did a rotation on dermatology. The instructor stated that 95% of dermatology can be learned in a two to three year residency program. It takes a lifetime to learn the other five percent. In internal medicine, in my opinion, one learns about 40% in the residency program; internists then spend the rest of their careers learning the other 60%.

This challenge to continue learning throughout my medical career was one I loved meeting. My love of learning started in the fourth grade at Hillcrest Elementary School in Morristown, Tennessee, where my teacher, Mrs. Murphy (her real name), taught us how learning could be fun. The desire to learn and the importance of learning have stayed with me ever since.

Through the years, in an effort to continue my medical education for the benefit of my patients, I have kept up with medical advances to the best of my ability. As will be mentioned in this chapter, I have been to many medical conferences and have regularly read much medical literature including the *Journal of the American Medical Association (JAMA), the Annals of Internal Medicine, The Medical Letter,* and others. Keeping up-to-date has been a huge help in making diagnoses for my patients. I have obviously made misdiagnoses but I remember those cases and consider *them* learning opportunities. These experiences have also taught me to have humility.

Over the years, I have had the privilege of going to many conferences at Johns Hopkins Hospital in Baltimore, Maryland. On two occasions, I attended the "Meet the Professor" series, extra courses that one can take for CME, or continuing medical education. At one of these courses, I had the privilege of meeting the physician who is known as the father of medical genetics. With that title, it is not surprising that this famous physician, Dr. William McKusick, was also a proponent of the human genome project.

As an extracurricular activity, Dr. McKusick led interested conference attendees on a tour of the historic old hospital during a "Meet the Professor" session called "Trip to the Dome." He brought us into the entrance of the hospital where we viewed "The Divine Healer." This fourteen-foot high statue of Christ is a replica of the original, sculpted in 1820 in Rome by the Danish sculptor Bertlel Thor Waldsen. Professor Stein, a sculptor and director of the Danish Royal Academy of Arts, made the replica. After its completion in 1896, it was dedicated at Johns Hopkins in the fall of that year. This statue had an important influence on my life as a person and a physician. Afterwards, we visited Dr. William Osler's office where he worked as the hospital's first chief of medicine. We then proceeded up the many series of stairwells to the cupula, or "the dome," on top of the hospital. There, Dr. McKusick pointed out famous landmarks in Baltimore, including Fells Point and the nearby harbors. It was quite humbling being in such a world-renowned academic medical center with such a famous physician. At the same time, I felt proud to *be* a physician while being in the presence of great doctors! After going to Johns Hopkins Hospital for a week of CME courses, I always felt inspired to come back and go to work knowing that the knowledge I had gained would help me to be a better physician for my patients.

As mentioned elsewhere in this book, making the correct diagnosis is the most important part of good medical care. William Osler himself advocated for the importance of the correct diagnosis but Osler was obviously aware that physicians are only human and capable of making mistakes. There is a story about Osler that Dr. McKusick shared with us. It went something like this. There was a man admitted to Johns Hopkins Hospital with what appeared to be a mass in his pelvis. Dr. Osler told him that he probably had a tumor such as a sarcoma. He was told to go home and live out his remaining time. However, he recommended that he be seen by a surgeon first. The surgeon saw the patient and performed a physical examination. He then placed a catheter into the patient's bladder. With drainage of the bladder, the mass disappeared! The patient went home happy. Dr. Osler, a self-deprecating man and a man with a good sense of humor, was able to laugh at his misdiagnosis of an obstructed bladder, particularly since the patient was unharmed.

Misdiagnoses unfortunately also occur with *bad* outcomes for the patient. Doctors dread these outcomes. Remember the comparison of medicine and baseball? I well remember a patient from Mississippi who came to the VA Hospital in Memphis where I was a resident. Jud Baker was a poor farmer who had raised seven children. He came in with abdominal pain. I remember his writhing around in pain on the examining table. Routine studies, as well as an ultrasound of the abdomen were non-revealing. He was later transferred to the GI, or gastrointestinal, service at the hospital. He underwent an endoscopy (a procedure where a tube with a light on it is placed through the mouth and into the stomach for diagnostic purposes) that was also non-revealing. Unfortunately, he died a few days later of a missed ruptured abdominal aortic aneurysm.

When I was a fellow in general internal medicine and on call for another doctor, a patient whom I had never actually seen called me at three o'clock one morning. In a few hours, he was scheduled to board a plane to Boston where he was to have a procedure at one of the Boston hospitals. He said he had been diagnosed with a hematologic disease but said he had a hemorrhoid that he wanted me to examine for him in the ER before his trip. I told him that the doctor in the emergency room would see him first. I emphasized that he should go, and told him I would be available if needed. Unfortunately, however, he did not go the ER. The following day, I heard that he had collapsed when he arrived at the airport in Boston. Taken to the hospital, he was found to have a perirectal abscess instead of a hemorrhoid. He died of sepsis with septic shock associated with the perirectal abscess. I felt a cold chill that day that I feel again even as I write these words. The words of Hippocrates are haunting, "Primum non nocere," or "First do no harm."

One of my patients, an older lady, was admitted to the hospital with fever and abnormal liver enzymes. There did not seem to be any evidence of infection. Lymphoma was the suspected diagnosis. A liver biopsy was performed that was completely normal. Over the next several days, her fever continued, despite multiple antibiotics. She died with no diagnosis. Her husband granted an autopsy. She was found to have Hodgkin's lymphoma. Older age is usually a negative risk factor for many types of Hodgkin's disease, so it was not at the top of my diagnostic list. The peculiar aspect of this case was that at the time of autopsy, her liver was chock-full of tumors! How could a biopsy needle have missed all those tumors? Strange, indeed!

Another elderly lady whom I had been seeing for hypertension had also had some visual complaints. Referral to her ophthalmologist revealed a finding in her optic disk (the point of entrance of the optic nerve into the retina) that was consistent with polymyalgia rheumatica-temporal arteritis spectrum of disease. Temporal arteritis is a disease of the elderly characterized by headache of which this patient did not complain. The headaches are usually in the temple, the location of the temporal artery. These patients can also experience visual symptoms and a feeling of being ill, like having influenza without the respiratory symptoms. In addition, the sedimentation rate is characteristically very high in this disease. This disease responds dramatically to steroids. If left untreated, it can lead to blindness in the affected eye.

She had received no steroids at all because I did not suspect temporal arteritis due to the absence of the characteristic headache. As a result, she had some vision loss. Afterwards, my suspicions were raised and on doing a sedimentation rate, hers indeed was very high. Needless to say, I felt bad about her loss of vision.

This patient had actually presented with temporal arteritis forme fruste. In medicine, forme fruste refers to the atypical presentation of symptoms and signs. I well remember a case of temporal arteritis presented in a medical journal. The typical patient with temporal arteritis is white and elderly with a high sedimentation rate. This particular patient was a 26-year-old African-American who had presented with a headache. His sedimentation rate was normal! However, he had a reddened appearance to an obviously enlarged temporal artery. A subsequent biopsy proved temporal arteritis! The astute physician must be on guard for such atypical presentations of disease.

These cases emphasize that physicians are human and make mistakes. In fact, I believe that one will find only one type of physician who does not make a mistake – the one who never does any patient any good.

As stated before, I learned "humility" from these patients. I will always remember the statue of Christ at the entrance to the old Johns Hopkins Hospital. At its base are the words from Matthew 11:28, "Come unto ME all ye that are weary and heavy laden and I will give you rest." The right great toe of Christ is shiny and worn from thousands of people having touched it over many decades.

These words are at the entrance to a hospital that today is at the forefront of patient care, education, and research. I believe these words are meant for everyone. In this case, it applied to not only the patients who were there to receive medical care but also to the physicians and all the medical staff who carried the responsibility of making the right diagnoses and caring for the patients who entered the doors of their hospital.

I have mentioned William Osler many times throughout this book. Known as the "father of modern medicine," he was at Johns Hopkins Hospital in Baltimore, Maryland, for many years. Dr. Osler was also known for bringing medical students out of the lecture hall to bedside clinical training. He established the first residency program for specialty training of physicians. Osler himself wrote of humility. He penned,

"Acquire the art of detachment, the virtue of method, and the quality of thoroughness, but above all the grace of humility." As a practicing physician, I have learned through the years that humility is one of the skills of an experienced physician. Indeed, if practicing medicine makes the provider more arrogant or more dogmatic, that provider has at once lost a great skill – that of practicing both the science and the art of medicine.

Despite missed diagnoses, these patients still took a lot of time. With these patients, however, I never felt I was running behind. With new insights into their problems and with a fresh "coat" of humility, with each patient I was, indeed, running ahead.

Chapter 17

"The Queen"

A wise physician said, "The best medicine for humans is love." Someone asked, "If it doesn't work?" He smiled and answered, "Increase the dose."

— Author Unknown

Up to this point, this book has been about the patients and my relationships with them. This chapter, however, is different. It is about Renee.

Renee Smith (her real name) worked with me as my nurse for 22 years and 3 months in Kingsport, Tennessee. She became a friend and trusted colleague with whom we shared the experiences of helping thousands of patients with their medical problems. She had a Hawkins County, Tennessee, work ethic. This, combined with good genes and Christian upbringing from her parents, as well as good training in school, was a great recipe for someone who would spend her life dealing with sick people. She was a woman of God, a wife, a mother to two baseball-playing boys, and a dedicated nurse (in that order) who always gave her best for the patients. Work was not just work for her. To those around her, it was her ministry.

Patients experienced a comfortable atmosphere that put them at ease when Renee greeted them with her warm smile in the waiting room or in her office. She treated patients and their families like friends. They would generally inquire about her two sons, whose pictures were proudly and prominently displayed in her office. On occasion patients would ask me about "the children." In later years, I would reply that my children were grown and doing fine. They would then correct me and say, "I don't mean your kids. I was talking about Renee's!" They even extended their love of her to her family whom they did not even know!

Renee worked part time for a while and, of course, took vacations. In her absence, another nurse filled in for her. The questions about Renee's absence were constant. "Where is Renee? Is she sick? Why is she not here?" The barrage of questions from patients became quite time consuming. Of course, I knew and appreciated that it simply showed their great admiration and love for her.

One particular day stands out prominently. Renee had a day off. I was helping an octogenarian with a cane get on the examining table. Halfway up onto the table he inquired about the whereabouts of Renee. Almost ready to fall, he would not sit down properly until he heard that indeed Renee was fine and was without illness or personal problems. Even at the end of the visit, he asked, "Well, when will she be back?"

Her relationship with our patients was strengthened by her frequent calls giving them lab results or referrals, or answering their many questions. With these calls, she demonstrated her genuine concern for their well-being. She did this to help the patients, not to please her superiors or me. Renee had a mind of her own, and she was pretty tough. She stood "tall" on taking the moral high ground and keeping the patient and their problems in the forefront.

Renee was the greatest nurse ever in getting the patients back to the examining room on time. This was very valuable as it gave me more time to interact with the patient. Once at a meeting of the providers the question was asked what the major obstacle was in seeing patients on time. The most frequent answer was that their nurse was not getting the patients back on time. I was perhaps the only doctor in the room who had the totally opposite experience with my nurse, Renee

"The Queen" was the nickname by which Renee was lovingly known by everyone in our office. From my point of view, it was a title fittingly bestowed. She knew how to get things done. On the other hand, if a patient came by for a concern or a chat, she willingly stopped her necessary duties and happily helped them with their problems. Her informing me of a problem that a patient perhaps did not want to discuss with me allowed me to approach that problem with the patient from a different perspective. When she told me about patients who could not financially afford the visit, including those who had no health insurance at all, I could then "adjust" their charge. Renee also had great rapport with all her "subjects." Sorry! I meant her co-workers! In addition, she was a very bright woman. I have given her as many as five tasks to do at one time. They would be completed well and in good time even without having to write them down. There were several times when data about a patient was pending. I would simply forget that a laboratory report or x-ray was not back yet. In her diligence, Renee might remind me weeks later that she had found a report about which I had previously forgotten.

Renee did add humor to our office. There is a sign in her office that read, "Nurses call all the shots around here." She was good about keeping me informed of our patients who passed away. As was our custom, we would then call the patients' families. On one occasion, she informed me about a patient with multisystem failure who had died, so I called the family. The patient's daughter answered the phone and informed me that her mother was fine and feeling the best she had felt in some time! We could have said that she had been resurrected as a result of good medical care. Instead, Renee and I had a good laugh about it! Apparently, there was an obituary of another person with the same name in the paper that day! From that time onward, we correlated obituaries in the newspaper with birthday records at the office.

Renee became part of the backbone of my practice for all those years. I owe a great deal of the success of my practice to her. This and my genuine admiration for her as a longtime friend and co-worker is the reason a whole chapter is devoted to "The Queen". She was my colleague in every sense of the word. Her modest demeanor and humility do not allow her to accept this compliment easily.

Even as I neared retirement, Renee played prominently in patient care. Many patients sent me letters of appreciation for my care of them. One lady even said that she has been seeing me for twenty years but that it had felt like forty years! I had to ponder that comment for a while. One particular note in the letters of appreciation was, "Dr. Reed, I hate to see you retire, but Renee – she can NEVER retire!" Another note from a couple stated, "Dr. Reed, we have always liked you as a doctor, but we LOVE Renee!"

Renee gave patients a big dose of medicine that all of us need. Part of the remedy for depression, bad news, anxiety and many physical problems was simply love exhibited through her concern, diligence, and ever-present smile.

The chapters in this book are about the humanity of the patient and their diseases. My time spent with patients, as stated, had always put me behind with my daily schedule. Because of her diligence, Renee ran behind, too. Renee always did her best to keep me running *ahead* in terms of time whenever possible. In addition, because of the patients' initial interaction with Renee, by the time I saw them in the examining room there was a sense of calm that had already begun to ease their fear, pain, unhappiness, or worry over their serious complaints or diseases. Her contribution to her profession cannot be counted in monetary terms. Her successful ministry will live in the hearts of patients, their families, and me for many years.

Chapter 18

Miracles

"Every cubic inch of space is a miracle."

— Walt Whitman

We often hope for miracles when something bad happens to us or our family or friends. While I have always believed in miracles, I often wondered why so many bad things happened to my patients. Upon looking into this early on, mainly through church-related activities such as attending and teaching Sunday school, my understanding of this idea began to grow. Rabbi Harold S. Kushner's book *When Bad Things Happen to Good People* taught me a great deal. His book taught me that sometimes bad things happen, and when they do, God is there as a source of *comfort*, not judgement. More answers came later in my studies with the reading of *The Will of God,* the sermons of Leslie Weatherhead, a minister in London.

I learned from the book of Job in the Old Testament of the *Bible* about the subject in some detail. In an effort to help Job understand the horrible loss of his family and property, his wife and friends told him that he had obviously done something terribly wrong that displeased God. In the end, however, Job learned that a person just has to *trust* God through times of suffering and hardship. There was no logic behind why the bad events had happened to him but by trusting and leaning on God instead of blaming Him, he got through those bad times.

This story points to one reason I think medicine and theology are so closely intertwined. One cannot find the answers to these questions through science and the practice of medicine alone. The answers can best be found by looking at these questions through the lens of theology (the study of God).

In the end, of course, there are no absolute answers for every patient who has something bad happen to them. However, I believe that every physician must develop some paradigm to help guide them in caring for the suffering. This paradigm does not provide answers for the physician but becomes a guide. I found mine in the church and its teachings.

One of the blessings in my life has been witnessing miracles. I have witnessed the great strides in medicine of seeing fewer people have heart attacks and strokes. This has resulted from improved lifestyles and better medications for high blood pressure, high cholesterol, and diabetes. In my early career, I witnessed many fewer amputations as a result of better controlled diabetes. When people have heart attacks and strokes, there are better interventions with coronary and carotid stenting. Metastatic lung cancer, breast cancer, and melanoma patients now live longer due to advances in immunotherapy and chemotherapy.

A miracle, like beauty, is often in the mind of the beholder, as I have discovered. Mrs. Gladys Berry, from Coeburn, Virginia, was a long-standing patient of mine. On one occasion, she called the office to say that a local Virginia doctor had diagnosed her with lung cancer. She had always been a non-smoker. About ten percent of lung cancer occurs in nonsmokers and can be associated with environmental factors such as radon, industrial pollution, and exposure to secondhand smoke. When she came to my office, she brought her chest x-ray with her. Indeed, it showed a very large mass in the right upper lobe of her lung. Careful inspection of this x-ray showed that the name on the x-ray was *not* Gladys Berry. I repeated her chest x-ray at our local hospital only to find out that it was completely clear. I informed her of the mistakenly labelled x-ray. As I suspected, she was delighted, expressing her feeling that God had clearly cured her. In the future, Mrs. Berry and her family often talked of her "cure" from lung cancer.

I had taken care of Ms. Phoebe Donaldson for about twenty years. Despite her diabetes and hypertension, she had done well through the years. One day, however, she came to the office with a cough, shortness of breath, and a headache. She was hospitalized and treated for pneumonia. However, her headache persisted, and she eventually lost consciousness. When she became unconscious, a spinal tap, or lumbar puncture, was performed. This is a procedure in which a needle is introduced into the spine between the lumbar vertebrae in order to examine the spinal fluid. She was indeed found to have meningitis.

She was put on a ventilator, during which time her blood pressure remained low. One weekend I had to be away from the hospital. On Friday, I decided to make some major changes in her medication. One of my colleagues saw her over the weekend for me. When I returned on Monday, she was alert, off the ventilator, had a good blood pressure, and was almost ready for discharge home! She was truly a miracle. In fact, from that time on, she became known as "the miracle lady". There have been such patients through the years although perhaps few as dramatic as Mrs. Donaldson.

In 1975, I was able to witness a miracle patient in the trauma unit of the John Gaston Hospital in Memphis, Tennessee. Although not an internal medicine patient as such, Mr. Willie Jones had been shot accidentally in the mouth with a 22-caliber gun. Examination showed no serious injury of the mouth or pharynx. Likewise, there was no neurologic damage at all. In addition, he had no injury to his windpipe (trachea), or to his esophagus. An x-ray showed a deformed 22-caliber bullet in the body of the second cervical vertebra. After full examination by multiple physicians and a tetanus shot, he left the ER.

I once heard a story about a man (not a patient of mine) who had suddenly lost the use of his legs for unknown reasons. Then, in about six months, he suddenly regained the use of them. All of us would proclaim this a miracle! However, as Walt Whitman might say in his famous poem *Miracles,* what a greater miracle it is that the rest of us have not lost the use of a leg to begin with. From this perspective, we all are witnesses to miracles happening all the time.

We are not able to have control over our own genetic pool. William Osler himself actually used the old adage that advises those who do not want varicose veins to be careful who they pick for grandparents since that trait is passed on through the generations. Also, while we have control over what we eat and how much we exercise, we have much less control over many environmental factors, such as pollution, the effects of global warming, second-hand smoke from parents who smoke cigarettes, and exposure to toxins such as asbestos in buildings and drinking water contaminated with lead, just to name a few. When I take into account the many thousands of diseases that we could have, every breath we breathe is a miracle.

Practicing internal medicine for over forty years has been a great joy and blessing in my life. In turn, I have learned a great deal about life itself as well as how miracles abound. I do hope that if patients remember me at all, it will not be because of my occasional tardiness. Having noted that, it has been a miracle that in my practice I was almost always "running behind."

Chapter 19

Frustrations in the Practice of Medicine: Acknowledging and Accepting Change

"Ships don't sink because of the water around them; Ships sink because of the water that gets in them. Don't let what's happening around you get inside and weigh you down."

— Author Unknown

Change is needed. Change is inevitable. With change, good may come. With change, bad results may also come. With change comes frustration.

The landscape of practicing medicine has indeed changed in the last forty years. Most of these changes have been good, especially with new medications, technology, research, and medical education.

Along with the above-named good innovations, there are also changes that have *not* benefited the patients or the practice of medicine.

I believe we are currently undergoing a transformation in medicine. Many of the changes that make up this transformation are having a negative effect on medical practitioners and their patients. While change is not easy for anyone to deal with, the frustrations accompanying these changes are felt because the good of the patient is not considered as the number one priority by the ones who are transforming medicine into a profit-driven business rather than a patient-driven mission.

Areas of change that have been a detriment to giving patients the best care possible are:

1. Insurance companies' greed and interference with the doctor-patient relationship
2. Profit-seeking by medical care delivery systems
3. Electronic health records

First of all, dealing with insurance companies has become a constant headache – a *bad* headache! The insurance companies do not have the best interest of the patients in mind. Mrs. Hanover's story below is a great illustration of this. Unfortunately, if the patient does not have a persistent advocate who can speak with the insurance company's representatives on his/her behalf, their decision as to whether or not to approve a provider's request may be based on the financial needs of the company rather than the medical needs of the patient.

Mrs. Norman Hanover was from Greeneville, Tennessee. She had risk factors for osteoporosis, including small stature, cigarette smoking, prior hysterectomy with ovary removal at an early age, and a mother who had osteoporosis with fractures. She seemed to be a poster child for osteoporosis but her insurance company denied coverage of a screening DEXA scan (a test that gives quantitation as to the degree of bone mineral loss, or osteoporosis). If payment for a patient's procedure, medication, etc. was denied, and the patient or physician wants to protest the decision, the insurance company requires the physician to contact them personally for "peer to peer" consultation. Because of this requirement, I made four calls to four different levels of consulting physicians who worked for the insurance company. All four denied my request. My fifth call was to the top level of a panel of consultants that had been convened in Memphis, Tennessee by the insurance company. Luck (or providence) was on my side this time. The panel was composed of mostly women. During the call, I discussed the importance of women's health and the fact that women are more than mammograms and Pap smears; *they have bones, too*! Women's bones are subject to fracture (as are the bones of men.) When the decision was made to approve Mrs. Hanover for a DEXA scan, I felt that I had won the lottery! I still feel good about it even today! As it turns out, however, her DEXA was only mildly abnormal. In addition, six months later, she changed insurance plans! So much frustration!

Secondly, the medical care systems (insurance companies, physicians, physician groups, health care companies, hospitals, pharmaceutical companies, durable medical equipment companies, etc.) are geared toward making a profit. While everyone likes to make money, the profit motive must *not* be more important than caring for the patient.

Balancing the ideas of making money and providing quality care for patients has always been a source of frustration. It has always made sense to me that I should give the best care I could give to the patients by applying my best diagnostic acumen along with other testing as needed. As a result, enough income would be generated to support my family.

In recent years, however, healthcare systems for whom medical providers work have put pressure on these providers to bring in *more* profit for the healthcare systems. They do this by requiring the providers to spend *less* time per visit with patients in order to see more patients per day. Of course, these actions can be detrimental to the patient because limiting the time spent with the patient decreases the emphasis on doing a thorough history and physical examination which is the backbone of a physician's practice.

Naturally, I believe that doctors should be paid well, especially considering all the years of college and training they have had. I do *not* believe, however, that the profit motive should supersede the primacy of patient care.

Financial toxicity, or economic hardship associated with the profit motive, is one of the outcomes for many patients. Some of those who are at the highest risk for being in this distressing situation are those who have serious and/or chronic illnesses or are victims of serious accidents. These seriously ill or injured patients may receive the best, highest quality medical care and even experience subsequent improvement. However, if that patient is unable to pay the copays or other expenses related to the treatments, he is more likely to experience "financial toxicity". Has he, in fact, received the highest quality care possible? No, the "toxin" of economic hardship has decreased the overall quality of the patient's care and treatment. Another way to look at this is that *cost* of medicine has become a *quality* factor in the practice of medicine. Remember that half of bankruptcies in the United States today are associated with medical bills.

My hope for the medical system is that it rewards the thoughtful, scientific practice of medicine – without regard to profit of the providers or systems. While I will avoid the politics of proposed payment systems, my one plea is to improve the avarice of the "profit motive" in medicine. Once again, while we all like to make money, making money should never be at the expense of the patient.

Thirdly, electronic health records (EHR) have also been a source of frustration. Originally mandated by the government and designed for better and more accurate record keeping, EHR initially seemed to be a good idea. Sharing of records among providers and healthcare institutions should have been a great asset in patient care. However, the various EHR systems simply do not "talk" to each other! Because of this, the *sharing* of healthcare data between providers and the subsequent effects of reducing duplication of testing, including imaging studies, have not yet been accomplished. EHR has proved to be of little value in increasing the quality of patient care in this way. In the last seven years, I have been a witness to and a participant in the EHR system. One of its problems is how *time-consuming* it is for providers who spend time on the computer that would be better spent with their patients. In the medical literature, constant attention is paid to EHR's part in the removal of the physician from direct patient care. Articles even appear from European countries about how resident training is interfered with by hours of computer work spent on EHR. In my own practice, I spent an average of two to three hours of extra non-face to face time per day away from patients because of dealing directly with EHR. Even worse, when the provider directs his attention to the computer while talking with the patient in the exam room, he is not able to adequately focus his attention on the history the patient is sharing with him and spends less time on the physical examination of the patient. As a result, a proper diagnosis is less likely to be made. In addition, when the provider spends time in the evening on the computer with EHR, he/she does not have time for reviewing patients with difficult problems (See "Diagnostic and Therapeutic Dilemmas", Chapter 13) or reviewing pertinent medical literature that can enhance the patients' care.

Another effect that time constraints have on the provider's face-to-face time with the patient is that the careful examination (the history and physical examination) of the patient is often being left out altogether. The history and physical examination forms the basis of good medical care by the physician. Lists of questions that the insurance company has decided are the most important ones to ask have often replaced this important examination.

Excellent medicine has far more to do with the patient as a person rather than as a person who has an electronic health record. Excellent medicine has to do with spending time with the patient. With this time, the medical provider can examine the patient and formulate a diagnosis. Later in the day, or in the evening, the provider can review patients who have difficult problems and review any pertinent medical literature. This thorough evaluation can reduce the need for extensive laboratory testing and imaging studies. Most importantly, rapport is established between provider and patient. This rapport helps to build trust which, in turn, strengthens the relationship. Discussions about personal problems, more intimate physical problems such as erectile dysfunction, advice about immunizations, and problems related to otherwise undiagnosed depression could all be more comfortably discussed. In addition, the physician comes to know the patient more closely. By spending time with my patients and getting to know them through the years, I have been able to remember patients' medical problems and medications just by seeing their face as I walk into the examining rooms. Spending hours of computer time on EHR limits quality face-to-face patient time that is so important in establishing good provider-patient rapport.

EHR has also become *a means for increased remuneration from insurance companies*. In other words, rather than being a *tool* to help in patient care, it has become an end in itself to enhance income. Unfortunately, EHR has now reached the height of importance in practices owned by large medical groups or medical corporations who have benefited financially from it.

I remember Mr. Homer Mullins from Kentucky who came often to see me, mainly about high blood pressure. He had anemia as well as a family history of colon cancer. I tried for a long time to have him undergo a colonoscopy to look for adenomatous polyps (precursor growths for colon cancer). I even wrote him a letter and called him at home about this. Colon cancer is a disease that no one should die from these days. Having a thorough history and physical examination by the physician along with testing such as a fecal Hemo-occult, colonoscopy, virtual colonoscopy (a CT scanning procedure), and the new DNA testing for cancer should preclude any future deaths attributable to this disease. Finally, one day Mr. Mullins told me, "Dr. Reed, I know that you're really concerned about my health. I'll get the colonoscopy." He did so and was found to have a resectable colon carcinoma (cancer that can be removed surgically) without evidence of any metastatic disease (spread of the cancer). Needless to say, I am not sure if he would have ever had the colonoscopy if I had only recorded it in the electronic health record that one was recommended. In fact, providers often record in the EHR that a colonoscopy or other test was recommended just to satisfy an insurance requirement when, in fact, the procedure was not even discussed.

Even though there were many frustrations in dealing with insurance companies, the profit motive, and EHR, I always tried to smile and keep the patient at the forefront of my mission as a doctor. I had to be willing to accept these changes at least to some degree. My own particular way of dealing with people, including patients, was forged when I was a young boy observing my father. Working as a salesman for a small bakery in Morristown, Tennessee, my father sold bread and other bakery products to the good people of Hancock County, Tennessee and Bell County, Kentucky. I rode with him on his route on many occasions and observed how he treated his customers with respect. He did his best to serve them with the best bakery products possible. As a result, he developed relationships that were part of his very being. By getting to know his merchants and their families, along with his being an honest, trustworthy salesman, he developed rapport with them. He became known as "the" bread man as opposed to "a" bread man. These relationships were constantly renewed by multiple visits over 51 years! This learning experience would later help me in developing relationships with *my* "customers," i.e., my patients.

In the mid-1960s, I was an orderly at Morristown-Hamblen hospital in Morristown, Tennessee. This was my first experience dealing with patients. Among other responsibilities, the job included giving enemas in preparation for barium enemas (a radiologic diagnostic test to look for colon lesions), as well as giving baths and inserting Foley catheters in male patients. Other tasks included working with traction devices for orthopedic patients and cleaning delivery rooms after vaginal deliveries in the OB suites. The opportunity to observe autopsies was memorable. The other orderlies and especially the RNs taught me a great deal about how to treat "the patient as a person" and about the importance of always putting the patients' interests first! Those important lessons learned by listening to their words and observing their actions stayed with me throughout my medical career.

Life is full of frustrations. They can weigh us down, keeping us from enjoying life to the fullest and from performing our jobs in the best way possible. One of my Physician Assistant colleagues in the Navy told me, "The best way to plow through the waters of the sea is to float with the waves." After all, the boat can be weighed down by the water that gets inside it and eventually causes it to sink. That is that same message that the unknown author shared in the quote at the beginning of the chapter. On the other hand, the sailors I worked with in the dispensary dealt with their frustration on the job by remembering the old Navy adage, "There's the right way, the wrong way, and the Navy way!" When a job had to be done, that adage helped to take the frustration out of the need to follow orders exactly as they were given and to get the job done. Working in this environment with these people helped me to see that everyone has frustrations and that people deal with their frustrations in different ways. In addition, frustration can lead to burnout, recognized for years now as a problem for physicians. Enriching the doctor-patient relationship by seeing the patient as a person rather than a disease gives the practice of medicine another dimension that can help to reduce burnout. This new dimension in their practice happens when the physicians recognize that the true importance of their work lies in helping people, not in dealing with the problems of medical care delivery systems.

These frustrations decrease the quality face-to-face time with patients that are necessary for good quality patient care. In addition, time with insurance companies, profit making, and the electronic health record took a lot of time. I found myself running behind constantly.

Chapter 20

Joys in Practicing Medicine: Home Visits

"Carve your name on hearts, not tombstones. A legacy is etched into the minds of others and the stories they share about you."

— Shannon Alder

One of the greatest joys in my practice of internal medicine was making home visits. Patients and families would literally open their hearts as well as their doors to me. I usually made these visits only when the patient was physically unable to come to the office at all. The patients I saw in the home had a myriad of diseases, including congestive heart failure, cancer, and stroke. Some were on hospice care. Most, but not all, patients who needed these home visits preferred to die at home as well.

The advent of hospice care in the last several years has been a great blessing in the lives of many people. Patients can now remain at home with family, have their caregivers, pastor, or the hospice pastor at their side, and usually do not have to worry about medical bills.

My memories of seeing patients in their home are many. It is such a blessing to have the following memories.

Mr. Roscoe Bush lived out in the country in northern Greene County, Tennessee. Incredibly poor in financial terms, he had earned a meager living by driving a truck and having a small farm. In his older years, his wife, Flossie, had developed severe dementia and was bedridden. Mr. and Mrs. Bush accepted my offer to see her in their home.

One cold February night after dark, Mr. Bush and I stood around his wood burning fireplace after I had examined his wife. He told me that he had always been a praying man and prayed to God daily about Flossie. Earlier in their life together, he and Flossie had struggled to make a living. At one point, there was not even any food in the house. He said he prayed to God for relief from his situation. The next morning, a truck carrying flour was going a little too fast around the curve on the road in front of his house. As a result, a sack of flour fell from the truck onto the road. He ran down to the road and picked up as much of the flour as he could. His family was thankful to God to have biscuits for dinner that day. As he finished his story, he told me that God answers all prayers. Flossie died a few weeks after my visit without unnecessary hospital, nursing home, or medical bills. The prayers of a loving husband were answered!

Mr. Max Baughn lived in Rogersville in an affluent neighborhood. He had dementia. When his wife Jean called to request a home visit, I went as soon as possible. Examination revealed that he had apparently had a stroke. He was still able to speak, but since he was elderly, I assumed that he might not be able to hear me very well. So I yelled at him, asking, "Mr. Baughn, how are you feeling today?" He said, "I'm fine but I'm not in the next county, you know!" I apologized to him and his wife. He lived a few more months after my visit and died without hospitalization, nursing home, or ambulance trips.

Mrs. Susan Hicks was a patient of mine while I was on staff at the University of Tennessee in Memphis, Tennessee. She had come to the office with problems of uncontrollable diabetes and diabetic peripheral neuropathy. One day, the family called and stated that Mrs. Hicks' leg looked infected. They stated that they would be unable to bring her to the office. After regular hours, I drove to see her at her home using directions from her son. Since I was from East Tennessee, I was less familiar with the Western side of the state, and smartphones with GPS had not been invented yet.

When giving me their address, they had not mentioned that they lived in Mississippi. After driving about thirty miles south of Memphis, I came to the Mississippi state line and got worried since I had no Mississippi medical license! I decided to keep going, and a few miles later, I found her house.

Upon my arrival, it was clear that she had evidence of cellulitis (infection of a bacterial nature) in her right leg, along with gangrene of her entire right foot. She refused hospitalization. Having expected to be treating a possible infection, I had brought a dose of an injectable cephalosporin antibiotic.

When I arrived back home, my odometer for the trip read 66 miles! I wondered how many other UT practitioners had driven that many miles for a house call! Soon after this, I moved to my own practice in East Tennessee. While I did not hear about her progress, I suspect that she did not do well.

Mrs. Florence Hartgrove lived in Church Hill, Tennessee. She had recently had a colostomy because she had an abdominal abscess following complications of diverticulitis (infection in a pocket or diverticulum in the colon or large bowel). This abscess occurred because of the diverticulitis presumably not being diagnosed early enough. At the time of my home visit, she was doing much better and had no fever or abdominal discomfort. The colostomy was functioning well. However, there was a problem.

Her family was very angry that she had had a colostomy that perhaps could have been avoided with an early diagnosis of diverticulitis. It seemed that all the bad events that had occurred were the fault of "you doctors." The family, though not the patient, expressed anger over Mrs. Hartgrove's circumstances. I explained to them that doctors are only human and that mistakes are made. I told them that after the diagnosis was made, we did the best we could to save her life.

Anger occasionally occurs with patients or their families because of medical mistakes or, more often, because of perceived mistakes. I have found it best just to listen to the complaints and to be sympathetic to their concerns. In these situations, I commonly expressed how sorry I was about their plight. Saying you are sorry does not equate with admission of guilt about medical events that may have transpired. Showing empathy generally tends to ease a tense situation. Responding defensively or with anger or resentment just increases their anger. In addition, I try not to explain or "educate" them about what really happened unless they ask specific questions. Additionally, if I see them months or years later out in public, I am friendly. In the long term, patients and families will remember you for your kindness instead of any defensive, angry, or resentful response.

Overall, it is more likely that your legacy as a health care provider will be imprinted on the hearts of patients and families because your kindness overshadowed any negative impressions they may have had about you. See the quote at the beginning of this chapter and Chapter 17, "The Queen."

There is a good story about a person's legacy, the source of which is unknown. A young minister arrived in a small town to pastor a church in the community. Before reaching the parsonage, his car ran out of gas. He had no money with him and no gas can, either. He walked to a service station a half mile down the road. The service station proprietor listened to his story but was unsympathetic, especially since the young minister had no money. The minister tried to be friendly and not to show resentment. As the conversation continued, the minister explained his reason for moving to this little town and shared that his grandfather had pastored the same church that he would be pastoring. Recalling his grandfather's name, the proprietor suddenly smiled and said he remembered him at that church when he was a young man. He said the preacher was the kindest man he had ever met. The proprietor then got a new gas can, filled it with gas, and drove the young minister to his car. What a legacy! By the way, the minister's grandfather had been dead for forty years. We as physicians and other healthcare providers would do well to remember this story of the legacy of kindness. I am sure the minister's grandfather had interactions with parishioners during which he would like to have reacted in a different way, but he chose kindness.

Making house calls did not really take time from patients in the office or hospital. I usually made them in the evenings or on weekends. However, they did cause me to be running behind in getting home to my family. This was especially true for the 66-mile trip to Mississippi!

Chapter 21

Medicine of Tomorrow

"The aim of medicine is to prevent disease and prolong life. The idea of medicine is to eliminate the need of a physician.

— William James Mayo

This chapter is mainly intended for those interested in making medicine a career – whether that career be as a physician, physician assistant, nurse practitioner or any allied health professional.

When the subject of the future of medicine is discussed, it is usually about technology, including new blood tests, new imaging, new surgical techniques, new medications, and new means of reimbursement for physicians and hospitals. However, my sincere hope is that the patient's best interest, not the amount of profit that can be made, will be at the forefront of any new treatment. Through the years, I have worked with medical students from the Quillen College of Medicine at East Tennessee State University. I was a volunteer assistant clinical professor of medicine. When they spent time with me in my office, I made sure they understood this concept. They also heard me discuss and demonstrate that putting the patient first is always paramount. As a primary care internist, one is uniquely suited to do this. I have taught the students that the physician must "sell himself or herself" to the patient, much as my father or any other salesman does. By doing this, a relationship forms that develops trust and rapport. However, there is a word of warning here; the rapport that is developed can never be used as a "marketing" tool or as a way to develop just a friendship with the patient. The rapport must be genuine and be a tool to enhance the trust between physician and patient.

By following the relationship-building list below, the provider-patient relationship can be enhanced and nurtured if used regularly. It may feel uncomfortable in the beginning but will become natural in time. These are the basic tenants of the practice of medicine learned by all medical students, but emphasized here.

1. The physician should always be standing to greet the patient in the examining room. An alternative is to accompany the patient from the waiting room into the examining room.
2. Shake hands with the patient and look him or her squarely in the eyes – always with a smile. Tell the patient that you are glad to see them and hope they are doing well. Then always sit down to take the history. Sitting instead of standing implies your intent to focus on them and to talk with them for as long as needed.
3. Inquire about the major problem. Then always allow the patient to discuss his or her complaints first. The provider's agenda is important but is always secondary to the patient's complaints.
4. Always allow the patient to enumerate all of his complaints. Do not interrupt him after even a half dozen complaints. You can always address the additional complaints at a later visit. Tell him or her that you will make another appointment for this purpose so he or she will know that you acknowledged their concern about the complaints.
5. Listen! Listen! Listen!
6. Write each of his complaints down if there are several of them.
7. Then ask this important question, "Is there anything else that bothers you?" This question lets the patient know that you have a genuine interest in him or her and are not trying to cut them off.

8. The past medical history should be reviewed in detail. If is the first visit for the patient, old records should be thoroughly reviewed. While this can be laborious, the patient will assume you will do this, especially if he brings a thick paper record or a CD full of PDF files. Often, important clues can be obtained from their previous evaluations. Ignoring old records can only lead to problems in the future.
9. The social history is an important part of the patient's story. It includes the patient's medications, smoking and alcohol history, use of drugs, including narcotics, occupational history, and travel history. The alcohol history is often neglected or minimized. (See Chapter 15.) The travel history is often neglected, as well. For example, if the patient has a fever, the provider would want to know if the patient had been to Africa and was exposed to some deadly virus, such as the Ebola virus. The social history may at times need to be focused, as well. For example, if a patient has fever and respiratory symptoms of an otherwise unknown origin, the physician should inquire about potential birds in the home, even including healthy parakeets. Without this detail, a diagnosis of psittacosis would NEVER be diagnosed.
10. Be sure to inquire about the family history. Important clues can be found that can help in the evaluation of the patient. I well remember the patient who had small muscles in his lower legs but had no complaints referable to them. His sign became more important when I learned that there was a family history of Charcot-Marie-Tooth disease (an inherited neurologic disease resulting in leg weakness).
11. The ROS, or "Review of Systems" is often left out of the examination. The ROS refers to important historical points that may have been left out in the initial interview. In this way, no history is left out that may become important later on. Unused by some

practitioners, it often becomes the secret to unlocking symptoms of diseases that may not present with obvious symptoms and signs until the diseases manifest themselves late term. I remember Mr. James Lighthouse from Church Hill, Tennessee, who had no complaints at all. However, on his review of systems, he reported occasionally having some blood in his bowel movements. He told me the blood was from hemorrhoids. Subsequent examination showed evidence of a positive stool Hemo-occult (test to look for otherwise unknown blood in the stool), but no hemorrhoids. He was referred for a colonoscopy and was found to have an ulceration at the tip of a polyp in the sigmoid colon (the lower portion of the colon just above the rectum). This ulcerated tip of the polyp turned out be cancer. In this case, the review of systems was instrumental in saving his life!

12. Then proceed with the necessary focused physical examination. The "laying on of hands" is a time-honored tradition that still has relevance. If time does not allow for physical examination of all their complaints, tell them that you will do this at a later date, perhaps with a return appointment in a week or month, etc. For example, I found it common that older patients would complain of memory loss. If this was at the end of a long list of complaints, I would schedule a return appointment in one month for a complete review and more detailed exam, including the MMSE, or mini mental status exam, and neurologic examination. The patient *must* be appropriately undressed and gowned before the examination. *Examination of the patient with their clothes remaining on* is *the equivalent of no exam at all!* The following cases are illustrative of the necessity of this recommendation. Mr. Douglas Smithfield was from Fall Branch, TN. He had come to see me for an examination after having seen another physician for several years. As with all new patients, I proceeded to do a

complete history and physical examination of Mr. Smithfield. He had been a previous cigarette smoker. He had no particular complaints except for a history of hypertension. As he got on the examining table and removed his shirt, he was noted to be short of breath. Examination showed wheezing on the left side of his chest. In addition, he had a markedly widened aorta on examination of his abdomen. A subsequent chest x-ray showed evidence of a mass in his left chest. It was subsequently proven to be lung cancer. An ultrasound of the aorta showed evidence of a large abdominal aortic aneurysm. He died six months later of metastatic lung cancer. On that first examination, he told me that I was the first doctor ever to have him remove his shirt. One week after Mr. Smithfield's first visit, his wife, Lois, came to see me. With her blouse off, I examined her breasts with a nurse in the room. She was found to have a mass in the right breast and was subsequently found to have widely metastatic breast cancer. She died six months later – two weeks after her husband's death. Mrs. Smithfield also commented that her previous doctor had never examined her with her blouse off.

13. Once rapport is firmly established, the trust relationship can be enhanced by being sure to have good communication with your patient. This is accomplished by being available, or at least having someone competent on call for you. Calling the patient occasionally is a good idea, as well. It is particularly good to communicate by email or letter about lab results. A call to the patient is mandatory when lab values or imaging studies are very concerning. As an example, when a woman had an abnormal mammogram, I called her myself.
14. Asking about other family members is an important part of the office visit. This is especially true if your patient has a spouse, parent, or child with a serious illness.

15. A favorite technique that I liked to use was to ask the patient to bring in an old picture such as a wedding picture or a picture of early military life. No matter how sad or worried a patient is about himself or a family member, they always smiled when I looked at the pictures and then commented, tongue-in-cheek, of course, "Why, you haven't changed at all!"
16. Calling the patient's family when the patient had died was my "last act of clinical significance" in my relationship with the patient. I have, on occasion, attended their funerals as well. It would seem that after years of visits and calls, the provider should make time for this one last call.

Remember – these points are to be used for the care of the patient and *not* as a marketing tool! *These sixteen points should be the foundation for the medicine of tomorrow*. While time-consuming, remembering to incorporate these time-honored points into the patient visit will insure that the provider keeps the needs of the patient as his/her highest priority. *All of these* points do not all have to be used at every visit but can be covered over a series of visits.

Ultimately, the practitioner must remember that clinical competence is the most important quality of the practicing physician. The good doctor keeps up with the medial literature, attends medical conferences, and reads constantly – always maintaining the sharpest diagnostic acumen. Making the right diagnosis and appropriate treatment plan is the most important task of the physician!

One of my favorite quotes that is apropos to the caring for patients is by John Dryden, England's first Poet Laureate. He wrote, "Errors, like straws, upon the surface flow; He would search for pearls must dive below." I hope in some small way that my forty years of practicing internal medicine has been consistent with this saying

The relationships built with these patients will be very satisfying to you in your practice years. It will help to reduce your potential for burnout by getting to know the whole patient as a person rather than just their disease. Your "family" becomes much extended and can help you learn to deal with your own problems by seeing how others deal with their problems. In addition, your own faith can be strengthened by hearing the many stories of disease and how it affects your patients' lives.

I am not sure if the need for physicians will ever be completely eliminated, the idea to which Dr. Mayo alluded. Like the poor, disease will always be with us. However, we can always do better to enhance good patient care.

Throughout the years, my desire to see each patient on time has seemed less important. If medical practitioners of the future will follow the above advice in their encounters with patients, they will perhaps be giving one of the greatest gifts they can give to their patients and the practice of medicine - time, or "running behind".

Author's Page

Dr. Richard K. Reed practiced medicine for over forty years. He graduated from the University of Tennessee College of Medicine, Memphis, Tennessee, in December 1974. After serving as a medical officer with the U.S. Navy at the Naval Weapons Center, China Lake, California, he returned to UT College of Medicine in Memphis to do a residency in internal medicine under Dr. Gene Stollerman. He was the first internal medicine resident at that institution to do a fellowship in general internal medicine. A Fellow in the American College of Physicians, he retired on March 31, 2019, after practicing medicine for 38 years in Kingsport, Tennessee.

www.ingramcontent.com/pod-product-compliance
Ingram Content Group UK Ltd.
Pitfield, Milton Keynes, MK11 3LW, UK
UKHW022018190726
13853UKWH00005B/1999

9 798629 550044